THE EVERYTHING.

DIGESTIVE HEALTH BOOK

Dear Reader,

When my father-in-law was diagnosed with colon cancer, the subject of digestive health suddenly hit home. Until then, I had been careless about my family's eating habits. After all, we rarely got sick—so why make waves?

We didn't eat much fast food, soda, or chips, and candy was a special treat, not an everyday occurrence. The more I learned, though, the more I realized I was gambling with my future, and that of my children. Just because nobody was sick didn't mean we were at our optimal health. Far too often, I reached for the frozen pizzas, white bread, mac-and-cheese boxes, and same three fruits over and over again. My grocery list looked the same from week to week.

I won't pretend it's been easy to change, and my girls sometimes look longingly at the processed food in the grocery store, but our diet is better than it's ever been. We introduce new foods every week and have found some we love. Pomegranate juice spritzer, anyone? We all want our families to be as healthy as they can today, and for a lifetime. It's not too late—good nutrition habits can start today.

Angie Best-Boss

Welcome to the EVERYTHING® Series!

These handy, accessible books give you all you need to tackle a difficult project, gain a new hobby, comprehend a fascinating topic, prepare for an exam, or even brush up on something you learned back in school but have since forgotten.

You can choose to read an *Everything®* book from cover to cover or just pick out the information you want from our four useful boxes: e-questions, e-facts, e-alerts, e-ssentials. We give you everything you need to know on the subject, but throw in a lot of fun stuff along the way, too.

We now have more than 400 *Everything®* books in print, spanning such wide-ranging categories as weddings, pregnancy, cooking, music instruction, foreign language, crafts, pets, New Age, and so much more. When you're done reading them all, you can finally say you know *Everything®*!

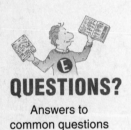

QUESTIONS?
Answers to
common questions

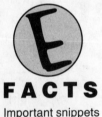

FACTS
Important snippets
of information

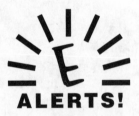

ALERTS!
Urgent
warnings

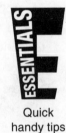

ESSENTIALS
Quick
handy tips

PUBLISHER Karen Cooper

DIRECTOR OF INNOVATION Paula Munier

MANAGING EDITOR, EVERYTHING SERIES Lisa Laing

COPY CHIEF Casey Ebert

ACQUISITIONS EDITOR Katie McDonough

SENIOR DEVELOPMENT EDITOR Brett Palana-Shanahan

EDITORIAL ASSISTANT Hillary Thompson

Visit the entire Everything® series at *www.everything.com*

THE
EVERYTHING®
DIGESTIVE
HEALTH
BOOK

What you need to know to eat well, be healthy, and feel great

Angie Best-Boss with
David Edelberg, MD

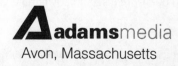

Avon, Massachusetts

An Everything® Series Book.
Everything® and everything.com® are registered trademarks of F+W Media, Inc.

Published by Adams Media, a division of F+W Media, Inc.
57 Littlefield Street, Avon, MA 02322. U.S.A.
www.adamsmedia.com

ISBN 10: 1-59869-959-8
ISBN 13: 978-1-59869-959-3

Printed in the United States of America.

J I H G F E D C B A

Library of Congress Cataloging-in-Publication Data
is available from the publisher.

This publication is designed to provide accurate and authoritative information with regard to the subject matter covered. It is sold with the understanding that the publisher is not engaged in rendering legal, accounting, or other professional advice. If legal advice or other expert assistance is required, the services of a competent professional person should be sought.

—From a *Declaration of Principles* jointly adopted by a Committee of the American Bar Association and a Committee of Publishers and Associations

Many of the designations used by manufacturers and sellers to distinguish their products are claimed as trademarks. Where those designations appear in this book and Adams Media was aware of a trademark claim, the designations have been printed with initial capital letters.

The Everything® Digestive Health Book is intended as a reference volume only, not as a medical manual. In light of the complex, individual, and specific nature of health problems, this book is not intended to replace professional medical advice. The ideas, procedures, and suggestions in this book are intended to supplement, not replace, the advice of a trained medical professional. Consult your physician before adopting the suggestions in this book, as well as about any condition that may require diagnosis or medical attention. The author and publisher disclaim any liability arising directly or indirectly from the use of this book.

This book is available at quantity discounts for bulk purchases.
For information, please call 1-800-289-0963.

Dedication

This project is dedicated to my mom, Sarah Sanderlin Houston, who forced me to write, encouraged me to make room for my writing, and continues to cheer me on. Special thanks to Rebekah Worthman, a wonderful editor/friend.

Acknowledgments

Special thanks to the International Foundation for Functional Gastrointestinal Disorders (IFFGD), the American Dietetic Association, the Crohn's and Colitis Foundation, and the George Mateljan Foundation, who graciously shared their time, resources, and expertise with me.

I am grateful to my agent, Bob Diforio, and editor, Katrina Schroeder, whose professionalism and expertise made writing this a pleasure.

Contents

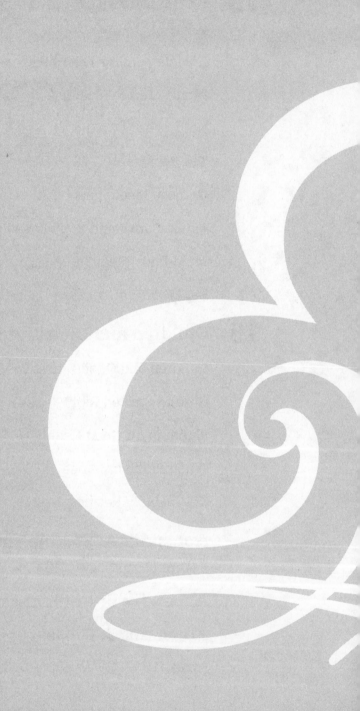

Top Ten Ways to Improve Your Digestive Health

1. Eat a balanced and varied diet that contains plenty of fruits and vegetables.

2. Choose foods that promote intestinal health like whole-grain breads and cereals, beans, dried plums, and nuts.

3. Limit fats and avoid concentrated sweets, emphasizing complex carbohydrates.

4. Get enough fluids by drinking 8 ounces with every meal or snack.

5. Give up caffeine.

6. Eat slowly and mindfully.

7. Don't eat before bed.

8. Exercise, doing activities you like.

9. Manage your stress.

10. Don't assume constipation, gas, or "upset" stomach is normal—it's a sign you need to make some changes.

Introduction

▶ ACCORDING TO THE NATIONAL Institutes of Health, more than 90 million Americans suffer from digestive disorders. From upset stomachs and heartburn to life-threatening cancers of the esophagus, liver, pancreas, and colon, digestive health problems account for as many as 35 million doctors' office visits a year.

Poor digestion can result in more than a stomachache or gas. Digestion is the machine that powers the body—converting food into a usable form of energy that is used in turn to create health and vitality. When that process doesn't go smoothly, the effects can be devastating. Digestive health problems can range from mild discomfort to excruciating pain. Chronic diarrhea or constipation can be debilitating and isolating.

Asthma, arthritis, allergies, and even cancer are all directly related to our digestive system health. What you feed your children and what you make for dinner can have a significant impact on long-term health. The good news is that the power is in your hands to make changes. Your digestive health is impacted by what you buy, by how you cook, by the chemicals you ingest, and by the way you move, sleep, work, and play.

Even people who maintain a healthy lifestyle get sick. There are no guarantees, but the choices you make can reduce your chances of digestive health problems. Plus, you can learn how to catch problems early enough to be treated. Only half of adults who should be screened for colon cancer have been screened. Why? Almost everyone has heard horror stories about how painful the test can be and how miserable it is to prepare for. The truth is, knowing exactly what to expect can help, and this book has all the information and encouragement you need to make that appointment you've been postponing.

To make matters more difficult, it isn't easy to discuss digestive health, even with physicians. Patients are often too embarrassed to acknowledge their concerns, and may suffer silently while experiencing daily abdominal pain, diarrhea, nausea, flatulence, and even incontinence. While this book doesn't replace the advice of a physician, readers can begin to take appropriate steps to make changes in their lifestyle and diet, and in the habits that are adversely affecting their health.

The book provides helpful tools so readers can assess their digestive health, keep a symptom diary, know when and how to find a gastroenterologist, and even tips on how to prepare for GI testing. Part of what makes this book so user friendly, and what's missing from other digestive health books, is the inclusion of 100 recipes. Parents learn their children need a high-fiber diet, and they are given a batch of kid-friendly, high-fiber recipes to get them started. When readers learn about the affects of caffeine on digestive health, they may decide to kick the habit, and having a handful of energy-boosting recipes will help make this is a book they turn to again and again.

It is possible to make changes in diet and lifestyle that can significantly improve indigestion, gas, bloating, and constipation. Feeling uncomfortable after eating, or having to plan outings with restrooms in mind, is not normal for our bodies. Sometimes, we have felt so bad for so long that we have forgotten what is was like to feel good.

It isn't too late to make changes. Whether you are retired or a new parent, the choices you make today will affect how you feel tomorrow and next month. Protecting your digestive health is important. It just might save your life.

Chapter 1

Assess Your Digestive Health

When it comes to overall wellness, maintaining your digestive health is just as important as maintaining your heart health, bone health, and the health of the rest of your body. Most people who are in good digestive health don't regularly experience symptoms like heartburn, gas, constipation, diarrhea, nausea, or stomach pain. Learn what normal digestive health looks like and why you shouldn't ignore those "gut feelings."

Importance of Healthy Digestion

To understand why digestion is so important, you must first understand the digestive process that occurs in your body. When you digest food, it is broken down into nutrients, which feed your body and keep it working well. Your body is made up of billions of cells. Like tiny building blocks, they work together to form every part of you. Cells make up your skin, bones, muscles, and organs. Your body uses nutrients to fix damaged cells and make new ones. Nutrients give cells what they need to work, grow, and divide.

Digestion begins in the mouth, where food and liquids are taken in, and is completed in the small intestine. The digestive system supports the human body. It is composed of a series of organs that break down and absorb the food you eat so that the nutrients can be transported into the blood stream and delivered to cells throughout the body.

Most people ignore our digestive system unless there's a problem. They rarely consider the role it plays in our overall health. To think, move, work, and learn, you need your digestive system to process your food and help utilize the nutrients. Your skin, hair, and even sleep can be affected by whether or not everything is working correctly.

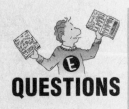

QUESTIONS

How common are digestive troubles?
During any particular day, almost everyone has gastrointestinal symptoms of some kind. Nearly half (46 percent) of Americans say digestive problems affect their day-to-day lives.

Your Intestinal Health Matters

People with poor digestive health might struggle with their weight, experience irregularity, nausea, bloating, constipation, stomach pain, diarrhea, heartburn, or gas on a routine basis. Poor digestive health also can prevent people from sleeping, working, exercising, or socializing with friends.

We know our digestive system is working properly when it can process important nutrients through the GI organs. The gastrointestinal organs include the stomach, intestine, liver, pancreas, and gallbladder. What does a normal GIS system look and feel like? If you have good digestive health, you should be close to a normal weight and go days without experiencing symptoms like heartburn, gas, constipation, diarrhea, nausea, or stomach pain.

When you have diarrhea and feel like you can't get too far away from a bathroom, or when you're dealing with constipation and feel uncomfortable no matter what you do, then your whole life suddenly revolves around your digestion.

Overall Health Impact

If you have poor digestive health, you might experience it in ways you never imagined. The Center for Disease Control (CDC) reports that 35 percent of cancer deaths result from dietary risk factors.

Poor diet and digestive health may be related to:

- Bad breath
- Heart disease and high blood pressure
- Reflux esophagitis (GERD)
- Crohn's disease
- Arthritis
- Osteoporosis
- Ulcerative colitis
- Psoriasis and eczema
- Chronic fatigue syndrome
- Asthma

How the Digestive System Works

When you eat things like bread, meat, and vegetables, they are not in a form that the body can use as nourishment. They must be changed into smaller molecules of nutrients before they can be absorbed into the blood and carried to cells throughout the body. Digestion allows your body to get the nutrients and energy it needs from the food you eat.

Parts of the Digestive System

The digestive system consists of the digestive tract and other organs that assist in the digestion process. The digestive tract is made up of organs joined together in a long tube that runs from the mouth to the anus. The digestive tract includes the following:

- Mouth
- Esophagus
- Stomach
- Small intestine
- Large intestine
- Rectum
- Anus

Other organs aid in the digestion process but are not part of the digestive tract. They include:

- Tongue
- Glands in the mouth that make saliva
- Pancreas
- Liver
- Gallbladder

Other organ systems, such as the nervous system, are also involved in processing food.

Starting the Process

It's time for breakfast. You get your bowl of cereal and take a bite. You chew and swallow. What happens from the moment the food goes in your mouth until it leaves your body? When you see, smell, taste, or even imagine a tasty snack, your salivary glands, which are located under the tongue and near the lower jaw, begin producing a digestive juice called saliva. Your teeth break the food into smaller pieces and the digestive enzymes in your saliva start to break down some of the carbohydrates. When you're ready to swallow, the tongue pushes a tiny bit of chewed-up food called a bolus toward the back of your throat and into the opening of your esophagus, the second part of the digestive tract.

You swallow by choice, but once the swallow begins, the digestion process becomes involuntary and moves along under the control of the nerves. The esophagus is like a stretchy pipe that's about 10 inches (or 25 centimeters) long. It moves food from the back of your throat to your stomach.

Muscles in the walls of the esophagus move in a wavy way to slowly squeeze the food through the esophagus. Think of it like squeezing toothpaste out of a tube. It would work even if you were standing on your head! A muscular ring called a sphincter allows food to enter the stomach and then squeezes shut to keep food or fluid from flowing back up into the esophagus.

The Stomach's Job

Digestion continues when food reaches your stomach. The stomach has a stretchy wall covered with special cells. Some of the cells make digestive juice to continue breaking down food. Some things you drink or eat like water, salt, sugars, and alcohol can be absorbed directly through the stomach wall. The rest needs the help of the stomach before passing down to the small intestine.

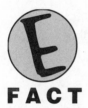

An adult's stomach has a volume of just ⅕ of a cup (1.6 fluid ounces) when it is empty, but it can expand to hold more than eight cups (64 fluid ounces) of food after a large meal.

Mucus coats the food and the wall of the stomach and helps protect the stomach wall from acid. Acid plays an important role in helping to kill germs in the food and soften the food. The stomach stores the swallowed food and liquid, which requires the muscle of the upper part of the stomach to relax and accept large volumes of swallowed material. Acting like a mixer, the lower part of the stomach mixes up the food, liquid, and digestive juices produced by the stomach by muscle action. Every twenty seconds, the muscles in the stomach wall squeeze and turn your dinner into a soupy liquid.

Next, the stomach empties its contents into the small intestine to convert food into absorbable nutrients and energy. Food moves, a teaspoon at a time, out of the stomach and into the small intestine. The amount of time it takes for the stomach to empty depends on the type of food being digested and the amount of fluid in it. The more fluid you have, the faster the stomach empties.

The Small Intestine and Liver

From the stomach, food enters the small intestine. The twenty-two-foot-long small intestine is a narrow tube that loops around your stomach several times and is the longest part of your digestive system. It does the bulk of the digestive work. It takes one to four hours for the small intestine to break food down into nutrients and absorb it into the blood.

A number of important digestive hormones and digestive enzymes help to regulate digestion, especially in the upper gastrointestinal tract. The small intestine is a coiled tube made up of three sections—the duodenum, jejunum, and ileum. It is covered with billions of microscopic, finger-like bumps called villi. The walls of the villi are very thin and covered with tiny blood vessels. The nutrients go through the walls of the villi and into your blood.

Blood carries absorbed nutrients through the bloodstream to the liver. The liver cleans the blood, straining out nutrients when they arrive. Some nutrients are stored in the liver and stay there until the body needs them. Other nutrients leave quickly and are distributed to other parts of the body. After every useful, digestible ingredient other than water has been wrung out of the remaining material, called chyme, the remaining waste passes into the large intestine.

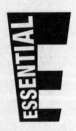

The intestine has a big job. More than a gallon of water containing over an ounce of salt is absorbed from the intestine every twenty-four hours.

Bile from the gallbladder (hidden just below the liver) and liver (located under the rib cage in the right upper part of the abdomen) emulsify fat and enhance the absorption of fatty acids. The enzymes in the pancreas cause chemical changes that, with the help of bile, break down proteins, fats, and carbohydrates. An enzyme is a protein that can cause chemical changes in organic substances like food.

Getting Rid of Waste

The undigested material from the small intestine is vegetable roughage (cellulose), meat connective tissue, some digested but unabsorbed nutrients, and large amounts of water. What's left over in the small intestine gets passed to the body's waste-processing plant, the five-foot-long large intestine. The intestine forms a big loop that runs up your right side, across your middle and down your left side.

The walls of the large intestine are smooth on the inside with large colonies of bacteria. The bacteria act on the undigested waste and convert it into gases, acids, and vitamins. There are three parts of the large intestine: the cecum, the colon, and the rectum.

The cecum is a pouch at the beginning of the large intestine that joins the small intestine to the large intestine. This transition area expands in diameter, allowing food to travel from the small intestine to the large.

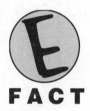

The large intestine is home to the appendix, the small fingerlike pouch that can become inflamed and be extremely painful. Some scientists suggest that the appendix—the slender two- to four-inch pouch located near where the large and small intestine meet, once thought to be worthless—may actually produce and protect good germs for your body.

The colon extends from the cecum up the right side of the abdomen, across the upper abdomen, and then down the left side of the abdomen, finally connecting to the rectum. The colon has three parts: the ascending colon and the transverse colon, which absorb fluids and salts, and the descending colon, which holds the resulting waste. Billions of bacteria live in the colon and help to ferment and absorb substances like fiber.

The rectum is the last twelve inches of bowel above the anus. Here, your feces wait to be excreted through the anus in your next bowel movement. The anus is held closed by a ring of muscles. When you have to go to the bathroom, you relax those muscles and feces are released from your body.

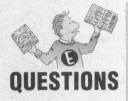

How long does it take for food to go through your digestive system?
It takes about twenty-four hours for a meal to move through your entire digestive system. The exact amount of time depends on the size of your meal and on the kinds of food you ate. In other words, soup moves a lot faster than a steak dinner!

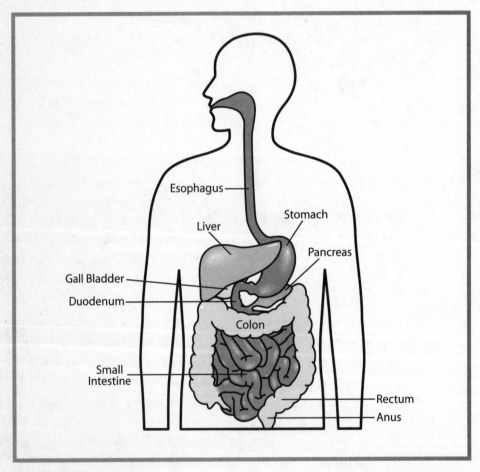

Esophagus

Liver

Stomach

Pancreas

Gall Bladder

Duodenum

Colon

Small Intestine

Rectum

Anus

The Digestive System

Create Good Digestive Health

Now you know how your system works. What's next is to discover all of the things you can do to promote good digestive health. The GI system has some pretty intricate architecture that makes it both sensitive and responsive to environmental changes.

Take Care of Yourself

Taking good care of your body will have a dramatic impact on the overall health of your digestive system. Your digestive tract is impacted by everything from the amount of sleep and exercise you get to your state of mind. If you get enough sleep, you allow your body time to repair tissue damage and get rid of waste. Exercise helps improve muscle tone and your mental state impacts how you digest and absorb nutrients. There's a lot you can do to improve your digestive health.

Choose Meals Carefully

Your meals, especially over a day or several days, should be balanced. That means having neither too much nor too little of anything. You need some fat because it slows down your intestinal tract, allowing slow-absorbing nutrients to be absorbed. But as you know, too much fat isn't good for any of our body systems. A well-planned meal allocates about 30 percent of its calories, or energy, as fat.

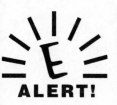

Maintaining good dental health is an important part of digestive health. The primary function of your teeth is to tear and chew food, to reduce it into smaller pieces. But if your teeth or jaws hurt, you will be less likely to eat a wide variety of healthy foods—especially fruits and vegetables.

There should also be many different foods in your diet. Eating a good variety of foods is the best way of ensuring you get all the nutrients you need. You know food contains important vitamins like A, C, E, D, and B complex, as well as essential minerals like zinc, chromium, calcium, and magnesium, but there are also hundreds of micronutrients—nutrients that are required in lower quantities but are nonetheless essential to keeping your body's intricate systems functioning properly. Plus, eating different things each day will keep you from getting bored and, hopefully, less likely to give in to the easy gratifications of junk food.

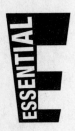

To boost variety in your diet, wander the grocery story aisles and find new things you never considered cooking, or find a unique fruit or vegetable at the farmer's market. If you eat the same fruits and veggies all year, you will miss out on the flavor and nutrients of eating produce when it is in season.

Get Regular Medical Screenings

You will learn a lot in this book about how to make lifestyle changes, add dietary supplements, eat well, and feel better. However, even if you embrace all of these changes, you still need to learn about what screenings you should have and when. Seeking appropriate medical care is another avenue to maintaining good digestive health.

It's Your Decision

When your digestive system is working the way it should, your body converts food into energy and nutrition to build, repair, and sustain itself. In a lifetime, your digestive system will process about 23,000 pounds of food. It has a pretty big job to do and when it isn't working right, you feel it. Heartburn, constipation, and diarrhea can all make you feel uncomfortable, but they can also be signs that it's time to make some changes. Starting today, you can take responsibility for creating and maintaining your body's digestive health.

Assess Your Health

Good health begins with good digestive health. Having digestive health means you have the ability to process nutrients through properly functioning GI organs, including the stomach, intestines, liver, pancreas, esophagus, and gallbladder. Between 60 and 70 million Americans experience some sort of digestive health problem. Are you one of them?

Lifestyle Limits

One key factor in determining your digestive health is how it affects your lifestyle. Does your digestive health affect what you do? If it does, it's time to make digestive health a top priority.

According to the Digestive Health Organization, many people report that poor digestive health impacts their lifestyles to the point where:

- 34 percent feel uncomfortable in social situations
- 32 percent experienced an embarrassing situation
- 23 percent have been depressed and lacked energy
- 20 percent avoid work or social situations altogether
- Nearly 20 percent limit physical activities/exercise
- 17 percent experience heartburn or abdominal pain more than five times a month

Normal Digestion

If you are in good digestive health, you should not be severely under or overweight. Typical digestion does not include regular periods of heartburn, gas, constipation, diarrhea, nausea, or stomach pain. Researchers believe one of the best ways to maintain a healthy digestive system is to eat a nutritious diet.

Normal Colon Habits

When it comes to regularity, everyone's different. Although having one bowel movement daily is a good frequency for some, there are many healthy people who have several movements daily and some who have as few as one every three to four days. The goal is to be symptom-free—that is, no pain, abdominal discomfort, bloating, constipation sensation, or heartburn.

Signs of a poorly functioning colon include:

- Straining to pass your bowel contents
- Having a hard stool that sinks to the bottom of the toilet
- Chronic diarrhea, loose stool, or constipation
- Excess gas, bloating, and abdominal cramping

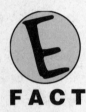

Download the Digestive Health Diary from Senekot (*www.constipation advice.co.uk*) to monitor and record your digestive habits.

When Something Isn't Right

Good digestive health may be defined by the absence of symptoms of functional gastrointestinal (GI) disorders. The Rome Multinational Working Teams (Rome II) has classified more than twenty functional GI disorders related to any of five anatomic regions: esophageal, gastroduodenal, biliary, bowel, and anorectal. These disorders may vary in their symptoms and causes, all are characterized by chronic or recurrent symptoms attributed to the gastrointestinal tract.

When the digestive system is out of balance, symptoms may include:

- Bloating, belching, burning, and flatulence after meals
- A sense of fullness after eating
- Indigestion, diarrhea, constipation
- Rectal itching
- Weak or cracked finger nails
- Dilated capillaries in the cheeks and nose in the nonalcoholic
- Postadolescent acne or other skin irritations such as rosacea

- Iron deficiency
- Chronic intestinal infections, parasites, yeast, and unfriendly bacteria
- Greasy stools
- Skin that's easily bruised
- Fatigue

Look Before You Flush

It may seem gross, but your stool can give you clues about your overall digestive health. The color of your stool, for example, can be indicative of digestive health problems. It should be the color of tan cardboard. Pale stool can be caused by some medications or a lack of bile. If your stool is green and you aren't eating lots of spinach, it could be that food is passing through your body too quickly and you aren't absorbing the nutrients you need. Black and red stools can be produced by some foods, medications, and artificial colors added to foods. Black stool can also indicate bleeding in the upper digestive tract.

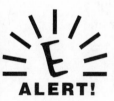

Unless you have been chowing down on beets or red velvet cake, the proper response to any deep red or black stools is an immediate check-in with your health care provider.

Your stool should also float. Bowel movements that sink to the bottom of the toilet may indicate too much protein and not enough fiber in your diet. The consistency of your bowel movement should resemble toothpaste. Pellet-like stools that are difficult to pass are signs of insufficient fiber and water.

Types of Digestive Problems

There are two basic types of health problems—functional, also called physiologic (no disease present), and organic, also called pathologic (symptoms caused by disease). If no pathologic changes can be found in the organ, the symptoms are regarded as annoying but harmless. Most health complaints are described as functional, which means no known associated organic or pathological tissue changes can be found by the physician.

Functional Digestive Problems

Functional gastrointestinal disorders are a group of disorders, including irritable bowel syndrome (or IBS), gastroesophageal reflux disease (or GERD), and chronic constipation or diarrhea. These extremely common conditions all have chronic or recurrent gastrointestinal symptoms that appear for at least twelve weeks within a year. Besides the symptoms, no structural or biochemical causes are found. The only way you can learn if you have a functional disorder is by visiting a health care provider.

Pathologic Digestive Problems

Organic digestive health problems are caused when there is a structural problem with a part of your digestive system. For example, a duodenal ulcer is an actual, visible sore on the inside lining of the first part of the small intestine (duodenum) that goes into the stomach. It is a structural abnormality and therefore an organic digestive problem.

Risk Factors for Digestive Problems

Whether the condition is functional or pathologic, there are a number of factors involved in how well someone's digestive system functions. A person's lifestyle—including diet, exercise, smoking, and alcohol consumption—is one of the key indicators. Someone's personal history is important as well. For example, if you have already had a bout with cancer, you are more likely to battle it again. Likewise, family history and genetics also play a role.

Just because you have one or more risk factors doesn't mean you will definitely develop poor digestive health. Knowing your risk factors to your digestive health can guide you into making the best choices for yourself—whether it's making lifestyle changes or learning symptoms you should be concerned about. Regular medical checkups and timely screenings are important for everyone, regardless of the number of risk factors.

Keep a Food/Symptom Diary

Even people with no digestive problems can benefit from keeping a food diary for two to three weeks. An honest look at what you eat (including portion size) could be a helpful resource in choosing how to improve health. Most people think they eat better than they do. Few people need to keep a permanent track record of everything that goes in their mouth, but after a few weeks, most people can see where healthful changes can be made. If you are not eating a healthful diet, sharing the diary with a doctor or nutritionist could yield helpful results.

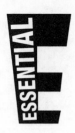

If you're ready for a high-tech food diary, try the free Tweet What You Eat, which uses a service called Twitter. Tweet What You Eat allows you to keep an itemized food diary using your cell phone and/or instant messenger service. Not only will it keep track of what you're eating, but it'll keep track of the times you eat too. To get started, just create your own free account at *www.twitter.com*.

Identify Culprits

For those with less than perfect digestive health, keeping a food and symptom diary can make a big difference in understanding what's happening physically. It can help identify troublesome foods and can serve as an important source of information for your doctor and nutritionist. Many patients are surprised to find that foods they didn't suspect were problems were actually symptom triggers. Do an online search for free food diaries to find a printable form that works for you.

Track Food/Beverage Intake

Here are some key things to look at when tracking your intake:

- **How much:** For this portion of your food diary, record the amount of food you ate. For example, list the number of items of food (12 pretzels) or the volume of that particular food (¾ cup) of bran cereal.

- **What kind:** In this portion of your diary, keep track of what food you ate—and you need to be as specific as you can. This includes everything from salad dressings to sodas, sour cream, sugar, and ketchup.
- **Time:** In this section, record the time of day you ate or drank.

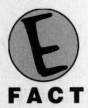

Create an online food journal by snapping photos with your camera phone. Some companies even offer professional diet coaching by reviewing your photos—no more cheating on serving sizes! If you use Twitter (mentioned earlier), you can even Tweet What You Eat during the day.

Track Feelings/Activities/Company

Also important in tracking what you eat is tracking where, with whom, and your mood when you eat.

- **Where:** It is important to note where you ate. Was it on the couch in the living room or in the car? At the kitchen table or inside a burger joint? Tracking where you eat will help you spot unhealthy patterns.
- **Alone or with whom:** You may eat differently (for better or worse) when you are with friends than when you are alone. Jot down whether you were alone or with family members or friends. Don't forget to list them.
- **Activity:** In this column, list any activities you were doing while you were eating (for example, working, watching TV, or ironing).
- **Mood:** Our moods can impact what we eat and how much. Describe how you were feeling—such as stressed, angry, worried, or excited—while you were eating.

Describe and Rate Your Symptoms

List any physical symptoms you may have before, during, or after eating and then use the following scale to rate the intensity of your symptoms:

- 0 = not severe
- 1 = mildly severe
- 2 = moderately severe
- 3 = severe

Chapter 2
Improve Upper GI Digestive Health

At some point, almost everybody gets heartburn—that uncomfortable burning sensation in your chest, the hot and bitter taste in your mouth. Twenty-five million Americans get heartburn every single day. You don't have to be one of them. Changes in diet and lifestyle as well as a fast-growing range of over-the-counter (OTC) and prescription medications can provide relief for most people. Learn what you can do to prevent heartburn, what your treatment options are, and when it is time to seek medical help.

Heartburn Hassles

The most common upper gastrointestinal complaint is heartburn. Heartburn is a burning discomfort that is generally felt in the chest just behind the breastbone. According to the National Heartburn Association, the burning sensation results when harsh stomach juices come in contact with and irritate the delicate lining of the esophagus, the tube-like structure that connects the mouth to the stomach.

These juices, which are produced by the stomach to help the body break down food, contain a powerful acid called hydrochloric acid. While the stomach is naturally protected from this potent acid, the esophagus does not share the same protective qualities as the stomach. So, if acidic stomach contents come into contact with the esophagus, its delicate lining can be irritated or injured and result in the sensation known as heartburn.

Heartburn Symptoms

While commercials may joke about heartburn, if you have it, it isn't funny. Heartburn can be uncomfortable and even downright painful. It can interfere with sleeping, with work, and, if left untreated, may lead to more serious problems.

Common signs and symptoms of heartburn include:

- Burning pain in the middle of the chest
- Sore throat
- Change in voice
- Vomiting and nausea
- Hiccupping and belching
- Difficulty swallowing
- Taste of acid in mouth
- Trouble sleeping
- Recurrent sinus and ear infections

Heartburn Causes

According to the Mayo Clinic, when you swallow, your lower esophageal sphincter (LES) a circular band of muscle around the bottom part of your esophagus, relaxes to allow food and liquid to flow down into your stomach. Then it closes again.

However, heartburn occurs when this valve relaxes abnormally or is not working properly, allowing stomach acid to flow back up into your esophagus. The acid backup is worse when you're bent over or lying down. When your esophagus gets hit by the stomach acid, it can be uncomfortable. It is also known as gastroesophageal reflux.

The most common causes include: hiatal hernia, pregnancy, obesity, and lifestyle choices. Obesity, for example, increases abdominal pressure, which can push stomach contents up into the esophagus. In some cases, symptoms disappear completely after an overweight person loses ten to fifteen pounds.

When Medications Are the Cause

Some medications can make heartburn worse by relaxing the lower esophageal sphincter (LES), allowing stomach contents to reflux back up into the esophagus. While they are likely to worsen heartburn, most medications will not cause heartburn in a healthy individual.

If you suspect that one of your medications may be causing heartburn, talk to your doctor. Keep track of when you began to experience these symptoms in addition to when you started taking any new medication. Never change or stop medication you take regularly without talking to your doctor.

Treating Heartburn

Occasional heartburn is common. But heartburn that interferes with your daily activities (like sleeping, exercising, working, and so on) should be evaluated by a physician. In some cases, a physician will require the patient to undergo testing, but most physicians will initially prescribe some form of acid-repressive therapy. If the patient does not respond to treatment, then it is more likely that testing will be required to make a diagnosis.

Making Lifestyle Changes

The most effective, and sometimes most difficult, way to improve your heartburn symptoms is to make lifestyle changes. Start with your diet—eat more fiber, consume less fat and sugar, and eliminate processed foods, caffeine, and alcohol.

Supplements

Some natural supplements may be useful in managing acid indigestion. Supplements that are thought to aid in reducing heartburn include the amino acid L-glutamine, vitamins C and E, and aloe vera. Some health care providers recommend taking a licorice extract known as DGL. Chewing DGL tablets may create a protective coating for the esophagus and stomach. Always talk to your health care provider about any supplements you are taking.

Keep a handle on your stress levels. The National Heartburn Alliance says 58 percent of frequent heartburn sufferers identify "hectic lifestyle" as a factor that contributes to their heartburn. While stress is a normal part of life, stress can lead to behaviors that may trigger heartburn—smoking, increased alcohol consumption, and so on.

Medications

For heartburn, you have several different over-the-counter and prescription medications that may provide relief. Your best option is always to make the lifestyle changes that eliminate the heartburn in the first place.

Antacids neutralize excess stomach acid. Even though stomach acid can still splash into the esophagus, it gets neutralized. Antacids provide fast relief of symptoms, but relief is short-lived, and usually lasts about half an hour.

Sodium bicarbonate is a simple treatment for episodic (or occasional) heartburn. Drink a solution of a small amount of baking soda mixed with water. The baking soda neutralizes the acid that causes the pain. Don't do this often, as excess sodium intake may raise blood pressure and cause other health problems.

H2 blockers are sometimes referred to as acid reducers or H2 receptor antagonists. They can be found in both prescription and nonprescription strength. Obviously, the prescription-strength formula is stronger than what you can purchase over the counter. They work by decreasing the amount of acid the body releases into the stomach. Acid reducers are known as systemic, which means they have to be absorbed into the bloodstream to work. The drawback of H2s is that they can take thirty minutes or longer before they start working. Because they don't offer fast relief of symptoms, H2s are better used to prevent heartburn. For example, if you are eating a late meal or something particularly rich that you suspect may causes problems, then taking an H2 may prove beneficial. Tagamet, Pepcid, and Zantac are all examples of H2s.

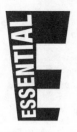

Over-the-counter medications are still medicines, even if they do not require a prescription. Follow the recommendations on the label and talk to your heath care provider about how often you are taking them, because antacids, for example, can interfere with other medications.

Alginates are another medication option and work faster than H2 blockers. Made from brown seaweed, alginates work by forming a protective barrier in the stomach. That barrier prevents stomach acid from refluxing back up into the esophagus. Because it is nonsystemic, it doesn't need to be absorbed into the bloodstream. Alginates provide heartburn relief for about four hours, which is longer than antacids. Because antacids work quickly, some brands of alginates offer both antacids and alginates in a single medication. An example of an alginate is Gaviscon.

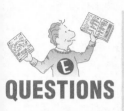

QUESTIONS

When is heartburn not just heartburn?
The pain caused by heartburn and heart pain (whether an actual heart attack or recurrent heart pain, called angina) can be so severe that both patients and doctors may have a difficult time distinguishing one from the other. Since there are all degrees of heart pain, your doctor may order additional tests to differentiate between the two diagnoses.

The most commonly prescribed medications for heartburn and GERD are the proton pump inhibitors, called PPIs. These are a class of medications that may work for people who do not respond to antacid or acid blockers. Brand names include Prilosec, Nexium, Aciphex, and Protonix, and, despite advertising to the contrary, they are all similar. Proton-pump inhibitors work directly to block acid production in the stomach cells. PPIs are systemic and work by deliberately disabling the system that controls the pH (acidity) of the stomach. Proton-pump inhibitors offer long-lasting relief, but do not work quickly.

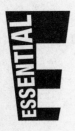

An easier method of raising your bed may be to use an eight- to ten-inch foam wedge underneath your mattress. Place a towel under your bottom and lower back to prevent you from sliding. Don't prop up your head with pillows—this crunches your stomach and may worsen reflux.

Heart symptoms include a feeling of fullness, tightness, or dull pressure or pain generally in the center of the chest. Pain may spread to the shoulders, neck, or arms and may be accompanied by a cold sweat; you might experience lightheadedness, weakness or dizziness, shortness of breath, and nausea and possible vomiting.

Nixing Nighttime Problems

Aside from all of the stomach pain and problems caused by GERD, many people also suffer from insomnia or lack of sleep because symptoms interfere with their nighttime rest. A survey of 500 adults conducted for AstraZeneca found that 91 percent had GERD symptoms that disrupted their sleep, and for 44 percent it happened at least once each week.

Raising the head of the bed uses gravity to keep stomach acid down where it belongs, in the stomach. Try raising the head of your bed four to eight inches by placing blocks or bricks under the legs. If your bed is on casters, try attaching jar lids to the blocks to cup the wheels and prevent your bed from rolling off the blocks in the middle of the night.

Heartburn Danger Signs

Many people think heartburn is uncomfortable but not a serious health problem. They're wrong. The American College of Gastroenterology says that frequent (occurring at least twice a week) unresolved heartburn can be serious. It's a symptom of GERD, a potentially serious problem. GERD is a severe form of heartburn which may be associated with esophageal ulcers, esophageal bleeding, narrowing of the esophagus known as peptic stricture, and even a premalignant condition known as Barrett's esophagus.

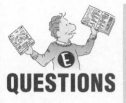

Is it true that smoking cigarettes is good for heartburn?
Not at all. Cigarette smoking exacerbates heartburn by relaxing the lower esophageal sphincter, the muscle between the esophagus and the stomach, which allows stomach acid to travel backward and enter the esophagus.

There are three causes of GERD: The esophagus's normal defenses are overwhelmed by the acid content of the stomach, the contents of the stomach are too acidic, or the food is not cleared from the esophagus fast enough.

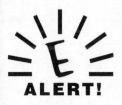

Hormone replacement therapy (HRT) may increase likelihood of developing GERD. A review of data on 51,637 postmenopausal women in the Nurses' Health Study found that HRT increases the risk of getting gastroesophageal reflux disease. Women who use selective estrogen receptor modulators—like tamoxifen for breast cancer and raloxifene for osteoporosis—also are at higher risk for developing GERD.

When to Seek Medical Treatment

Persistent and severe heartburn that isn't treated or comes back quickly with over-the-counter medicine may signal other problems. If your symptoms become worse, if you take medication longer than directed on the label or are having problems swallowing, then it may be time to seek medical attention.

Also there are a few foods that worsen heartburn and should be avoided, such as:

Foods
- Allspice
- Black pepper
- Chili peppers or powder
- Chocolate
- Cinnamon
- Citrus
- Cucumber
- Curry
- Fried foods
- Garlic
- Horseradish
- Mustard
- Nutmeg
- Onion
- Peppermint
- Radishes
- Sugar
- Tomatoes
- Vinegar

Beverages
- Alcohol
- Caffeinated drinks
- Carbonated drinks
- Coffee
- Grapefruit or orange juice (fresh-squeezed may be better)
- Nonherbal tea
- Tomato juice

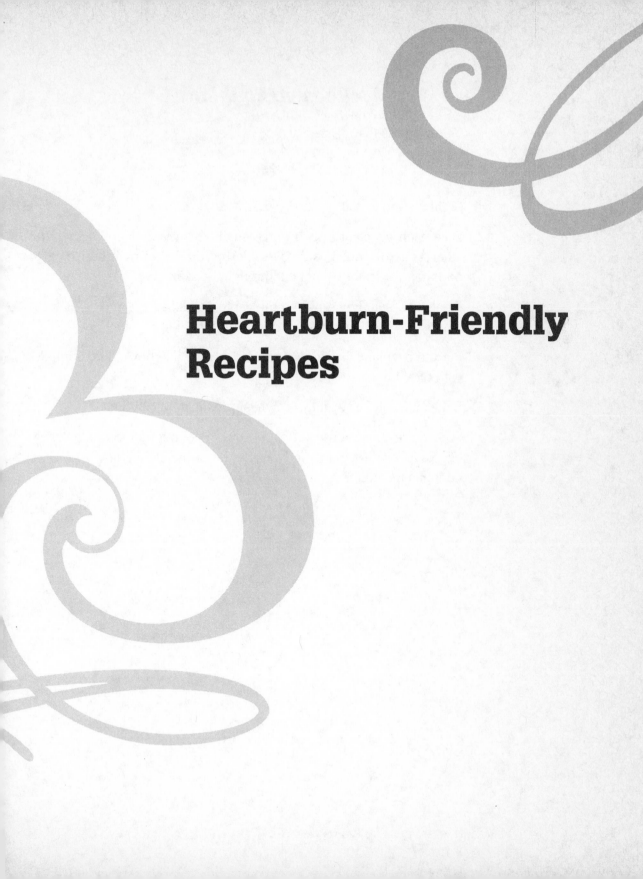

Heartburn-Friendly Recipes

Roasted Eggplant

Serves 4

Ingredients
2 eggplants
¼ cup fresh herbs that you can tolerate—such as rosemary, thyme, oregano
1 tablespoon minced garlic
1 tablespoon extra-virgin olive oil
2 tablespoons sesame seeds

Very small eggplants are the best but you can use larger ones.

1. Preheat oven to 350°F.

2. Slice each eggplant in two parts lengthwise. Make deep cuts with a small knife diagonally across the flesh, from left to right horizontally, and then vertically. Do not cut through the skin.

3. Finely chop all the herbs and the garlic and fill all the cuts of the eggplant.

4. Put the eggplants in an ovenproof dish skin side down, and sprinkle with olive oil.

5. Bake until soft and slightly brown, approximately 45 minutes.

6. Sprinkle sesame seeds over eggplant and cook for 2 more minutes. If eggplants get brown too early, cover the dish with aluminum foil and continue baking.

Basmati Rice, Butter Beans, and Pistachios

Red peppers are usually tolerated, but green and yellow peppers may create problems. If you are sensitive to red peppers, don't include them.

1. In a medium nonstick saucepan, heat oil on medium heat.

2. Add pepper, gingerroot, and rice, coating in olive oil. Stir in the water and lemon juice and heat until boiling.

3. Reduce heat to a simmer, cover and cook 15 minutes or until rice is done.

4. Stir in the butter beans and cook until heated through, no more than 5 minutes.

5. Stir in the mint and pistachios; serve warm.

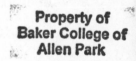

Serves 4

Ingredients

3 teaspoons olive oil
1 large red bell pepper, cut in thin slices
1 tablespoon gingerroot, grated
1 cup basmati rice
2 cups water
1 tablespoon lemon juice
1 (19-ounce) can butter beans, rinsed and drained
⅓ cup chopped mint
¼ cup sliced pistachios

Grilled Flank Steak

Cilantro contains an antibacterial compound that may prove to be a safe, natural means of fighting salmonella, a frequent cause of foodborne illness.

1. Mix all ingredients except the steak together in a large bowl. Separate out a small portion of the marinade for use later. Add the meat to the marinade.

2. Marinate 2 to 12 hours in the refrigerator, turning meat occasionally.

3. Cook on medium-high grill for 10 to 15 minutes on each side; as it grills, brush the meat with reserved marinade.

4. Slice meat diagonally across the grain and serve.

Serves 4

Ingredients

½ cup low-sodium soy sauce
¼ cup dry red wine
3 tablespoons vegetable oil
⅓ cup chopped cilantro
2 tablespoons chopped gingerroot
2 tablespoons Worcestershire sauce
Celery seed, (optional)
1–1½ pounds flank steak

Rotini Pasta with Broccoli and Canadian Bacon

Ingredients
16 ounces whole-wheat rotini
    pasta, uncooked
3 tablespoons olive oil
1 teaspoon minced garlic, as
    tolerated
1 (14.5-ounce) can reduced-
    sodium chicken or
    vegetable broth
1 tablespoon fresh basil, or 1
    teaspoon dried Italian
    seasoning
1 cup frozen broccoli
4 ounces low-sodium
    Canadian bacon
Grated Parmesan cheese
    (optional)

*You can easily substitute cooked chicken or turkey for the
Canadian bacon if you wish.*

1. Begin cooking the pasta according to package directions.

2. Heat oil over medium heat in saucepan. Stir in minced garlic, pour in the broth; stir in basil or Italian seasoning and cook until just boiling.

3. Place frozen broccoli in colander. Drain the pasta directly over the broccoli. Return the pasta and broccoli to the pan; pour in the broth.

4. Thinly slice and cube Canadian bacon.

5. On medium-high heat add the bacon to the pasta and toss well to combine. Cook for about 2 minutes, or until hot.

6. Serve with grated cheese, if desired.

Heartburn Alert
Tomato sauces frequently cause heartburn. When serving pasta dishes, use a light broth as a sauce.

Sweet Honey Apricot Chicken

*The enzymes in the honey aid in digestion of food,
especially raw sugars and starch.*

1. Blend honey, preserves, and ginger and brush mixture onto chicken.

2. Heat remaining mixture in small saucepan and set aside.

3. Grill or broil chicken about 8 to 10 minutes on each side until meat is no longer pink and juices run clear when pierced with a fork.

4. Glaze cooked chicken with warm honey mixture and serve.

Serves 4

Ingredients
2 tablespoons honey
3 tablespoons apricot
    preserves
1 teaspoon ground ginger
4 boneless, skinless chicken
    breast halves

Seasoned Oven Fries

*Since fast-food fries are out of the question, try a healthier version.
This recipe works well with sweet potatoes, although
you may want to experiment with the seasonings.*

1. Preheat oven to 450°F.

2. Toss potato wedges with oil, salt, and thyme (if using).

3. Spread the wedges out on a rimmed baking sheet.

4. Bake until browned and tender, turning once, about 30 minutes.

Serves 4

Ingredients
2 large Yukon Gold potatoes,
    peeled and cut into
    wedges
2 tablespoons extra-virgin
    olive oil
¼ teaspoon salt-free
    seasoning or sea salt
    (if tolerated)
¼ teaspoon dried thyme
    (optional)

Serves 4

Ingredients

1 teaspoon olive oil
1 cup red bell pepper,
    chopped
1 teaspoon dried Italian
    seasoning
2 cups spinach, coarsely
    chopped
⅔ cup water
1 (16-ounce) can navy beans,
    drained
2 cups fresh vegetable broth
    or 1 (14-ounce) can low-
    sodium vegetable broth
1 can no-salt-added tomato
    paste
½ cup carrots, fresh or frozen
1 (14-ounce) can quartered
    artichoke hearts, drained
½ cup canned or frozen corn
1 (9-ounce) package
    uncooked fresh cheese-
    filled tortellini
1 cup grated fresh Parmesan
    or Romano cheese

Tortellini, White Bean, and Veggie Soup

For extra flavor, serve this soup in warm bread bowls.

1. Heat oil in a large Dutch oven over medium-high heat.

2. Add red bell pepper and Italian seasoning and sauté 5 minutes, or until pepper is tender.

3. Add spinach, water, navy beans, vegetable broth, tomato paste, carrots, and artichokes, and bring to a boil.

4. Reduce heat and simmer for 30 minutes.

5. Add corn and tortellini and cook until thoroughly heated. Sprinkle with cheese.

Ginger Cake with Blueberries

Full-fat cakes are likely to disagree with you, but a light angel-food or sponge cake with fruit or nonfat ice cream is usually a safe bet. Change the fruit with what you have on hand or in season.

1. Preheat oven to 350°F.

2. Beat together the molasses, butter, egg, buttermilk, and ginger.

3. Stir in the flour. Dissolve the baking soda in a tablespoon of hot water, then add to the flour mixture. Fold in blueberries, mixing lightly.

4. Bake in greased and floured shallow square cake tins or muffin pans until cake tests done (about 35 minutes).

Serves 4

Ingredients
½ cup molasses
¼ cup butter
1 egg
½ cup buttermilk
½ tablespoon ginger
2 cups flour
¾ teaspoon baking soda
1 tablespoon hot water
1 cup blueberries

Cornbread Muffins

Often, cornbread has too much fat, but this recipe is adapted to be low-fat and good for you.

1. Preheat oven to 350°F.

2. Mix and sift dry ingredients.

3. Add buttermilk, egg substitute, and oil.

4. Pour into muffin tins that have been sprayed with nonstick spray.

5. Bake 20 to 30 minutes until golden brown on top.

Serves 8

Ingredients
1 cup yellow corn meal
½ teaspoon salt
½ cup all-purpose flour
1 tablespoon sugar
¼ cup ground flax seed
¼ cup wheat germ
2 teaspoons baking powder
1 cup low-fat buttermilk
½ cup egg substitute, beaten
1 teaspoon vegetable oil

Apple Snack Cake

Serves 16

Ingredients
1¼ cups boiling water
1 cup quick-cooking oatmeal, uncooked
1¾ cups all-purpose flour
¾ cup granulated sugar
¾ cup firmly packed brown sugar
½ cup wheat germ, any flavor
2 teaspoons baking soda
½ teaspoon ground nutmeg
1 teaspoon ground cinnamon
½ teaspoon salt
½ cup chopped nuts (optional)
2 cups peeled, chopped apples
⅓ cup no-sugar-added applesauce
1 ripe banana, mashed
1 egg plus 2 egg whites
1 teaspoon vanilla

Wheat germ is high in vitamin E, protein, fiber, polyunsaturated fat, vitamins, and minerals. Get in the habit of adding it to baked goods, cereal, and oatmeal.

1. Preheat oven to 350°F. Coat a 13" × 9" baking pan with nonfat cooking spray.

2. Combine water and oats in bowl and set aside.

3. In separate bowl, mix together flour, sugars, wheat germ, baking soda, cinnamon, nutmeg, and salt. Add nuts.

4. In oat mixture, add apples, applesauce, banana, egg, egg whites, and vanilla. Mix well.

5. Add dry ingredients to wet ingredients, mixing only until moistened. Do not overmix, or the cake will become dry.

6. Pour into pan.

7. Bake 40 to 45 minutes, or until a toothpick or wooden skewer inserted into the center of the cake comes out clean. Cool on wire rack.

8. As an optional step, sprinkle with confectioner's sugar.

Poached Pears and Raspberries

You can substitute other fruit, such as apples, peaches, apricots, or plums, in this recipe.

1. Combine the juices in a bowl, then slowly stir in the cinnamon and nutmeg.

2. Peel the pears, leaving the stems and removing the core from the bottom of the pear.

3. Using a shallow pan, stand pears in pan. Slowly add the juice mixture to the pears and turn burner to medium heat.

4. Without boiling, simmer pears for 30 minutes, turning the pears frequently.

5. When pears are soft, place them on individual dessert plates.

6. Spoon juice over pears, then garnish with raspberries. You may add orange zest or you may purée the berries in a blender and pour over pears. Sprinkle with sweetener if desired.

Serves 4

Ingredients
1 cup white grape juice
¼ cup apple juice
1 teaspoon ground cinnamon
1 teaspoon ground nutmeg
4 whole pears
½ cup fresh raspberries
2 tablespoons orange zest
Sweetener to taste

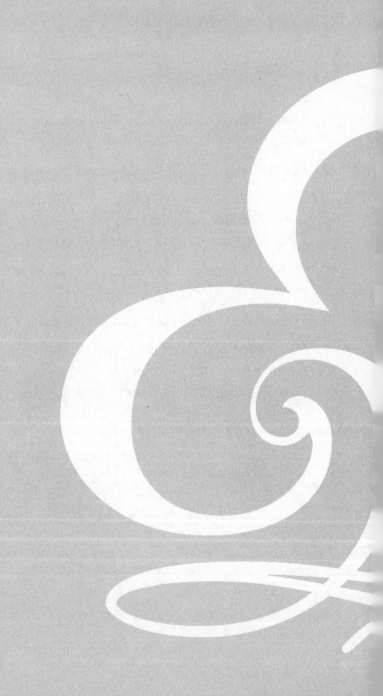

Chapter 3
Improving Lower GI Health

Lower gastrointestinal problems are not only uncomfortable, but they can also impact your quality of life. Diarrhea, constipation, and gas happen to everybody and they can be painful, frustrating, and embarrassing. Lower GI problems just aren't something people generally talk about, either with each other or with their physicians. Find out how to treat common lower GI problems, know when they require medical attention, and most important, learn what you can do to prevent them.

Dealing with Diarrhea

Diarrhea can be caused by food poisoning, bacteria, or bacterial toxins in food that you can pick up at restaurants, or eating food that has been kept too long. Gastrointestinal viruses can result in diarrhea and vomiting, but are fortunately also short-lived. Diarrhea is characterized by frequent trips to the toilet, a greater volume of loose, watery stools, and abdominal cramps.

Diarrhea Self-Care

The best way to treat diarrhea is to drink plenty of fluids, avoiding caffeine and alcohol. Try to drink four to six ounces of clear fluids every hour. Pedialyte or sports drinks are also good choices. Over-the-counter medications may help relieve the symptoms. Rest, and when you can begin eating, start with small amounts of bland food: broths, steamed vegetables, and boiled rice.

ALERT!

If you have HIV or AIDS, then you should contact your health care provider when diarrhea first begins. It is important not to wait until it gets worse or you become dehydrated. With a compromised immune system, you may be at higher risk for developing complications.

Seeking Medical Care

Diarrhea is very common and usually not serious. In fact, more than 90 percent of all cases of diarrhea are treated at home and do not need medical attention.

However, you should seek medical attention:

- If you are unable to tolerate any food or drink
- If you show signs of dehydration (dry mouth, headaches, weakness, dark urine)
- If you have a high fever and significant abdominal pain
- If you are elderly, or if the ill person is an infant or young child

- If have serious underlying medical problems, such as diabetes, or heart, kidney, or liver disease

Emergency Treatment

Go to the emergency room if you have severe diarrhea along with high fever, moderate-to-severe abdominal pain, or dehydration that cannot be managed by drinking fluids. If the diarrhea appears to contain blood (may be bright red or may look like black, thick tar), or if you are very sleepy or are acting unusual, then you need emergency care.

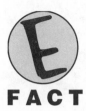

FACT

Diarrhea is a common side effect that people experience when taking antibiotics. Studies have shown that ingesting certain probiotics can substantially decrease incidences of antibiotic-associated diarrhea. Drinking two probiotic drinks a day is often enough too show benefits.

Diarrhea can be a symptom of underlying general diseases that are not specific to the gastrointestinal tract: diabetes, neurological diseases, liver diseases, gallbladder disease, and pancreatic disease. Diarrhea that lasts longer than a week or two needs the attention of your physician.

Coping with Constipation

More than 4 million Americans claim to be constipated most or all of the time. Some studies have estimated this number to be as high as 55 million, according to the American Gastroenterological Association (AGA)

Constipation Causes

Temporary, or acute, constipation is usually caused by a lack of high-fiber food, liquids, and exercise. Some common constipation causes include:

- Not drinking enough liquids
- Pregnancy

- Irritable bowel syndrome
- Lack of exercise
- Ignoring the urge to have a bowel movement
- Laxative abuse

Change Your Diet

As later chapters will explain in greater detail, your diet plays a major role in your bowel habits. Eating a high-fiber diet and drinking plenty of liquids are the easiest and most effective changes to make to eliminate constipation.

Constipation Self-Care

There are several natural products that you can take to relieve constipation. Magnesium is essential for relaxation of smooth muscles, including the large intestine, and it also can have a slight laxative effect. To add it to your diet, begin with 200 milligrams magnesium oxide or magnesium citrate every night. Until your bowels move regularly, you can increase the dosage in 200-milligram increments every few days. The dose for magnesium is individual, so begin low and increase the dosage as needed. Reduce the dosage if you experience loose bowels.

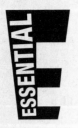

Daily consumption of certain probiotic fermented dairy products may have an effect on occasional constipation and can also help shorten long intestinal transit time, improving regularity.

Rhubarb root powder (Rheum officinale) is one of the safest and least violent irritant laxatives, but it should be reserved for occasional use only. Another natural treatment you can take is triphala. Triphala, an Ayurvedic remedy for regulating the bowels, is a combination of three fruits that tone the muscles in the large intestine. It should be used on a regular basis, however, and not just when temporary constipation occurs.

Medical Care for Constipation

See your health care provider if constipation has continued with no improvement for several weeks after changing dietary habits. If the person experiencing constipation is a child or an elderly person, call sooner.

Some medications can also cause constipation. If you take these medications and are having problems passing stool, talk to your physician:

- Pain medications (especially narcotics)
- Antacids that contain aluminum and calcium
- Blood pressure medications (calcium channel blockers)
- Antiparkinson drugs
- Antispasmodics
- Antidepressants
- Iron supplements
- Diuretics
- Anticonvulsants

Intestinal Gas

You may not realize it, but every single person gets intestinal gas. There are just two ways to eliminate it—burping or passing it through your anus. Not only does everyone have gas, we have more than we think. Most people create about one to four pints a day and pass gas about fourteen times a day. Where does it come from? There are a couple of sources. Swallowed air is one culprit as are byproducts from foods that are broken down and mixed with normal bacteria in the colon or large intestine. Colon bacteria is the culprit behind the unpleasant odor.

Some foods are known gas producers including:

- Beans
- Vegetables such as broccoli, cabbage, Brussels sprouts, onions, artichokes, and asparagus
- Fruits, such as pears, apples, and peaches
- Whole grains, such as whole wheat and bran
- Soft drinks and fruit drinks

- Milk and milk products, such as cheese and ice cream, and packaged foods prepared with lactose, such as bread, cereal, and salad
  dressing
- Foods containing sorbitol, found in some sugar-free candies and
  gums

Intestinal Gas Prevention

The less air you swallow, the less gas you'll pass. Make sure to exercise and keep tabs on what you eat, but some bad habits may make you uncomfortable. Things like smoking, gum chewing, sucking on hard candies, guzzling any-thing, and drinking carbonated beverages can add to your gas output.

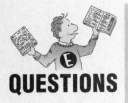

QUESTIONS

Can my dentures increase belching?
It sounds odd, but it's true. A pair of poorly fitting dentures can increase the air that goes down your gullet. And the more air that goes down, usu-ally comes back up.

You're likely to swallow more air when you drink from a bottle or use a straw than when you drink straight from a glass. If you tend to wolf down your food, you're taking in a lot of air as well. Eating slowly and chewing your food well cuts down on gas caused by air.

Doctors may prescribe prescription or over-the-counter medicines to help reduce symptoms. Digestive enzymes, available as over-the-counter supple-ments, help digest carbohydrates and may allow people to eat foods that nor-mally cause gas.

Hemorrhoids

Hemorrhoids can be either internal or external. Hemorrhoids are enlarged, painful veins in your rectum. They are like the varicose veins you might see on a person's legs. More than half of all Americans over age thirty will develop hemorrhoids at some time in their lives.

Causes of Hemorrhoids

Hemorrhoids can develop from any increase in pressure in the veins in the lower rectum. Common sources of pressure are constipation, diarrhea, pregnancy, obesity, and especially frequent straining with bowel movements. Eating a poor diet leads to constipation, which can cause straining on the toilet.

Hemorrhoid Prevention

Increase your fiber intake—especially whole ground flax seeds. Eat plenty of fruits, vegetables, and whole grains to help prevent painful hemorrhoids. If you aren't willing to make dietary changes, or dietary changes don't appear to be helping, then consider adding psyllium seed husks to your diet. They are available in a variety of forms in drugstores and health-food stores. Some people have success with an herbal mixture called triphala for constipation. From the Ayurvedic tradition, it can be purchased in capsules in health food stores. With any of these methods, follow the dosage on the label. Also drink plenty of water and get regular exercise.

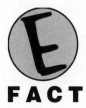

Many women experience hemorrhoids for the first time during pregnancy. The pressure of the fetus in the woman's abdomen, coupled with changes in hormone levels, cause the hemorrhoid vessels to enlarge, and during actual childbirth, the pressure on these vessels keeps increasing. These are usually temporary, and over-the-counter treatment is safe to use.

Hemorrhoid Self-Care

The swelling and pain of hemorrhoids can make life miserable. Over-the-counter lotions and ointments work for some people. Old-fashioned witch hazel is soothing and is fairly inexpensive. Another inexpensive treatment option is to sit in a sitz bath of warm water for ten to fifteen minutes. You can sit in the bathtub or in a special basin you place on top of the toilet. Make sure that the bath water is warm but not too hot, or it will irritate your skin even more. Adding ingredients like soap, Epsom salt, bath oil, or anything else may irritate the hemorrhoids.

Medical Treatment for Hemorrhoids

In some cases, hemorrhoids are very painful or they bleed excessively. When this occurs, medical treatment is necessary. Your treatment options vary, but include: sclerotherapy (where chemicals are injected into the hemorrhoids), infrared coagulation (a special device used to destroy internal hemorrhoids), banding (a rubber band is placed around and strangles the hemorrhoid), and hemorrhoidectomy (surgical removal).

Living with Inflammatory Bowel Disease (IBD)

Inflammatory bowel disease is the name of a group of disorders that cause the intestines to become inflamed (red and swollen). Crohn's and a related disease, ulcerative colitis, are the two main disease categories of IBD. Although it can involve any area of the GI tract from the mouth to the anus, it most commonly affects the small intestine and/or colon.

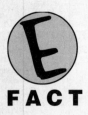

FACT

Some studies show a higher incidence of Crohn's disease and colitis in people who have had an appendectomy. Though the exact cause or causes of inflammatory bowel diseases are not known, it is possible that altered gut flora and genetics are critical to the development of these diseases.

Inflammatory Bowel Disease Causes

Investigators do not yet know what causes this disease and are looking at everything from genetics to the immune system to the environment. According to the Crohn's and Colitis Foundation, foreign substances (antigens) in the environment may be the direct cause of the inflammation, or they may stimulate the body's defenses to produce an inflammation that continues without control. IBD runs in families, so there is some genetic connection.

Inflammatory Bowel Disease Symptoms

IBD symptoms can be grouped into two categories. The first set of symptoms are those related to the digestive system:

Intestinal Symptoms of IBD
- Abdominal pain and cramping
- Bloating/distension
- Blood in the stool
- Loss of appetite
- Mucus in the stool
- Persistent diarrhea
- Ulceration in the digestive tract

Non-Intestinal Symptoms
- Delayed growth and sexual maturation in children
- Eye irritations
- Fever
- Fissures
- Weight loss
- Worsening of symptoms during menses

Get a Diagnosis

There is no single test that can establish the diagnosis of Crohn's disease with certainty. To determine the diagnosis, physicians evaluate a combination of information from the patient's history and physical exam. They examine the results of laboratory tests, X-rays, and findings on endoscopy and pathology tests, and exclude other known causes of intestinal inflammation. X-ray tests may include barium studies of the upper and lower GI tract.

Treatment Options

Because there is no cure, the goal of medical treatment is to suppress the inflammatory response. This accomplishes two important goals: It allows the intestinal tissue to heal, and it relieves the symptoms of fever, diarrhea, and abdominal pain. Once the symptoms are brought under control (this is known as *inducing remission*), medical therapy is used to decrease the frequency of flare-ups (this is known as *maintaining remission*, or *maintenance*).

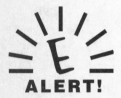

Pregnant women with inflammatory bowel disease have an increased risk of a premature birth or having a low-birth-weight baby if they have a flare up of the disease. Women with IBD recurrence delivered their babies at thirty-five weeks, on average, compared with almost thirty-nine weeks for women who did not experience a relapse. Talk to your health care provider if you have IBD and are pregnant.

Inflammatory Bowel Disease Self-Care

Living with a chronic illness like IBD can be very difficult and requires a great deal of support. As much as possible, lifestyle changes can be made to minimize the risk of inflammation. A healthy diet that restores needed nutrients, exercise as tolerated, and complementary care for psychological support are all necessary.

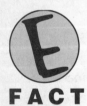

Researchers in the Netherlands report 22 percent of IBD patients in their study developed colon cancer before the starting point of screening recommendations. The researchers said screening should be based on patient risk factors, such as disease severity, age of IBD onset, and family history of colorectal cancer.

Living with IBS

Irritable bowel syndrome affects the large intestine and causes a host of problems including bloating, abdominal cramping, diarrhea, and constipation. It occurs when the intestines squeeze too hard or not hard enough and cause food to move too quickly or too slowly through the intestines. It is also known as functional bowel syndrome, irritable colon, spastic bowel, and spastic colon. IBS is not a disease—it's a functional disorder—and it's actually characterized as a brain-gut dysfunction.

IBS Sufferers

More than 20 percent of Americans suffer from IBS, which affects more women (75 percent) than men. Women may have more frequent symptoms during their menstrual periods.

Irritable bowel syndrome (IBS) does not have to rule your life. In fact, many people have symptoms mild enough so as not to disrupt their lives. In about a fourth of people diagnosed with IBS, work, school, and other activities are sometimes disrupted. At times, eating a specific type of food may trigger symptoms. For others, physical and emotional factors play a role, and stressful events may affect their symptoms.

Symptoms of IBS

IBS symptoms can very from person to person, and can vary in severity and duration in individual people. Typical symptoms include:

- Diarrhea
- Constipation
- Bloating
- Excess gas
- Abdominal pain
- Nausea
- Back pain

It's *Not* All in Your Head

One of the most common misconceptions about IBS is that it is purely a psychological problem. It isn't. It is a real physiological condition that can be mild and irritating or excruciating and life-changing.

However, IBS is made worse by stress. Stress can aggravate all kinds of medical conditions. For example, asthmatics can suffer from an asthma attack when they're stressed, and IBS patients can have an IBS attack when stressed. That doesn't mean that IBS is caused by stress any more than asthma is caused by stress.

Get a Diagnosis

The cause of irritable bowel syndrome isn't known, and getting a diagnosis can be difficult. In fact, IBS patients see an average of three physicians over three years before receiving a diagnosis. It used to be thought of as a diagnosis of exclusion. That is, it was diagnosed by ruling out everything else first. If nothing's left, it must be IBS. That is no longer true.

Because IBS is not a disease, diagnosis depends in part on determining whether or not your symptoms match those that have been medically established as definitive of IBS.

With the Rome criteria, you are believed to have IBS if abdominal pain or discomfort is continuous or comes and goes for a total of at least twelve weeks during the year, and two of the three following conditions occur:

- Pain is relieved by having a bowel movement
- The frequency of bowel movements changes
- The stools' appearance or form changes

Mistaken Identity—When It's Not IBS

Making a diagnosis of IBS can be difficult, and it is necessary to rule out other potential digestive health concerns. It can be helpful to know that these symptoms are not typical of IBS: pain or diarrhea that often awakens/interferes with sleep, blood in your stool (visible or occult), weight loss, or fever.

People with irritable bowel syndrome are statistically more likely to have upper GI problems (like GERD or reflux). However, they are not more likely to develop colon cancer.

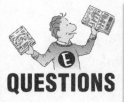

QUESTIONS

Where did the Rome criteria for irritable bowel syndrome originate? At the 13th International Congress of Gastroenterology in Rome, Italy, in 1988 a group of physicians developed a system to classify the functional gastrointestinal disorders based on clinical symptoms. Known as the Rome criteria, the guidelines outline symptoms and apply parameters such as frequency and duration to make possible a more accurate diagnosis of IBS and other digestive disorders.

IBS Self-Care

Many sufferers of IBS have found some of these tips to be handy:

- Eliminate all products containing carageenan (these include soy milk and ice cream).
- Take probiotics with meals; the friendly bacteria they contain can help stabilize the digestive tract.
- Take carob powder for diarrhea (mix a tablespoon with applesauce and honey). Used occasionally, this remedy can soothe irritated intestines
- Take peppermint oil if you have abdominal pain or cramping. Buy enteric-coated capsules and take one or two of them three times a day fifteen to thirty minutes before meals.
- Try slippery elm powder. Prepare a soothing gruel by combining one teaspoon of the powder with a teaspoon of sugar and two cups of boiling water. Stir well, flavor with cinnamon and drink one or two cups a day.

- Take 500 to 1,000 milligrams of turmeric a day. It is a powerful anti-inflammatory agent that treats inflammation of the gut at the microscopic level, another possible contributor to IBS.

Make Dietary Changes

No one diet will work for everyone with IBS, but there are some guidelines that may help. Any food high in fat, insoluble fiber, caffeine, coffee (even decaf), carbonation, or alcohol will create problems. Why? All of these food categories are either GI stimulants or irritants and can cause violent reactions of your gastrocolic reflex. These irritants directly affect the muscles in your colon and can lead to pain, constipation or diarrhea, gas, and bloating.

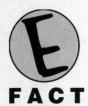

Many people with IBS find it is wise to completely eliminate all dairy products from their diet. Even if not lactose intolerant, dairy products can be a trigger for many people. Try rice milk substitutes for dairy.

Most IBS sufferers should eat a low-fat, high-protein diet and avoid these items:

- Alcohol
- Caffeine, found in coffee, tea, many carbonated drinks, and chocolate
- Nicotine, from smoking or chewing tobacco
- Dairy products that contain lactose (milk sugar), such as milk, cheese, and sour cream
- Spicy foods, including salsas or many ethnic foods that use chile peppers
- Foods high in acid, such as citrus fruit
- Foods high in fat, including bacon, sausage, butter, oils, and anything deep-fried
- Sorbitol and xylitol, artificial sweeteners found in some sugarless candies and chewing gum

Dietary Downfalls

Many people with IBS find it helpful to keep meals low in fat and high in carbohydrates. Carbohydrates include breads, pasta, rice, fruits, vegetables, and cereals. Some foods that you will be able to tolerate include:

Breads and Grains
- Whole-wheat flour, whole-wheat bread, whole-wheat cereal
- Wheat bran, whole grains, whole-grain breads, whole-grain cereals
- Granola, muesli, seeds, and nuts
- Popcorn
- Beans and lentils

Fruit
- Berries, grapes, raisins, and cherries
- Pineapple, peaches, nectarines, apricots, and pears with skins
- Rhubarb
- Melons
- Oranges, grapefruits, lemons, limes
- Dates and prunes

Vegetables
- Greens (spinach, lettuce, kale, mesclun, collards, arugala, water-cress, and so on)
- Whole peas, snow peas, snap peas, pea pods
- Green beans, kernel corn
- Bell peppers (roasted and peeled they're safer)
- Eggplant (peeled and seeded it's much safer)
- Celery, onions, shallots, leeks, scallions, garlic
- Cabbage, bok choy, Brussels sprouts
- Broccoli, cauliflower
- Sprouts (alfalfa, sunflower, radish, and so on)

Medical Treatments

While research continues, there is no medical cure for IBS. Treatment usually means making lifestyle changes (for instance, eliminating stress and trigger foods and adding relaxation techniques) and treating IBS symptomatically. The most recent new treatment for sufferers of IBS that manifests itself as chronic constipation is Amitiza, a medication that acts by increasing the motility of the large intestine.

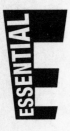

For more information about eating for IBS, visit Heather Van Vorous's website. The author of *Eating for IBS* offers encouragement and support for creating an eating plan that doesn't mean deprivation, never going to restaurants, bland food, or an unhealthily limited diet. Check it out at *www.helpforibs.com*.

IBS Recipes

Papaya Salsa

Serves 4

Ingredients
1 cup diced fresh mango
1 banana, sliced
1 cup diced papaya
3 tablespoons lime juice
1 tablespoon olive oil
1 teaspoon salt, or to taste
1 tablespoon chopped fresh
   mint

Look for a papaya that is firm and has a nice yellow color—not green. Cut a ripe papaya in half, scoop out the seeds, and cut into bite-sized pieces.

1. Toss together the fruit in a bowl.

2. Pour in the lime juice and olive oil.

3. Season to taste with salt, and stir to combine. Sprinkle with chopped mint leaves before serving.

4. Serve over rice, yogurt, or oatmeal.

Spiced Cranberry Apple Sauce

Serves 4

Ingredients
8 apples
1 cup cranberries
2 teaspoons cinnamon
½ teaspoon ground cloves
Ground nutmeg to taste

Large quantities of either cranberry juice or cranberry capsules may cause diarrhea in people with IBS.

1. Peel, core, and chop apples.

2. Place cranberries and apples in slow cooker.

3. Stir in cinnamon and cloves.

4. Cover and cook on low for 4 hours or until cranberries and apples are very soft.

5. Add nutmeg or brown sugar to taste.

Roasted Beets

To prepare beets for roasting, simply scrub the skin. Don't peel them or trim off the bottom. Remove the greens, but leave an inch or two of the stems to protect the color. Once the beets are cooked and cooled, pull off the skins.

1. Preheat oven to 400°F.

2. Wash beets, sweet potatoes, and carrots and cut into chunks.

3. In a bowl, toss the beets with ½ tablespoon olive oil to coat.

4. Spread in a single layer on a baking sheet.

5. Mix the remaining 2 tablespoons olive oil, garlic powder, salt, pepper, and sugar in a large resealable plastic bag. Place the sweet potatoes and carrots in the bag. Seal bag, and shake to coat vegetables with the oil mixture.

6. Bake the beets for 15 minutes in the preheated oven. Mix sweet potato and carrot mixture with the beets on the baking sheet. Continue baking 45 minutes, stirring after 20 minutes, until all vegetables are tender.

Serves 4

Ingredients
6 medium beets
3 medium sweet potatoes
2 large carrots
2½ tablespoons olive oil, divided
1 teaspoon garlic powder (if tolerated)
1 teaspoon kosher salt
1 teaspoon ground black pepper
1 teaspoon sugar

Grilled Lemon Salmon

Serves 4

Ingredients

1½ pounds salmon fillets
Lemon pepper to taste
1 tablespoon crushed
    rosemary or thyme
⅓ cup low sodium soy sauce
⅓ cup brown sugar (if
    tolerated)
⅓ cup lemon juice, fresh
⅓ cup water
½ cup vegetable oil or
    medium dry sherry

One four-ounce serving of wild salmon provides a full day's requirement of vitamin D and is a good source of omega-3 fatty acids.

1. Sprinkle salmon fillets with lemon pepper and rosemary.

2. Mix together soy sauce, brown sugar, lemon juice, water, and vegetable oil until sugar is dissolved.

3. Place fish in a large resealable plastic bag with the soy sauce mixture, seal, and turn to coat. Refrigerate for at least 2 hours, turning several times.

4. Lightly oil grill or skillet. Place salmon on cooking surface and discard marinade. Cook salmon for no more than 6 to 8 minutes per side, or until the fish flakes easily.

Lemon Root Vegetables

Serves 4

Ingredients

4 medium carrots
2 cups rutabaga (about 2
    medium rutabagas)
1 cup parsnips (about 2
    medium parsnips)
½ cup water
2 tablespoons butter or stick
    margarine (if tolerated)
1 tablespoon apple juice
    concentrate
1 tablespoon lemon juice
½ teaspoon grated lemon
    peel
¼ teaspoon parsley

You might not have cooked with parsnips before, but they resemble pale carrots and the flavor is slightly stronger. You can substitute them for carrots in many recipes.

1. Peel and cut vegetables into 3-inch julienne strips.

2. In a large saucepan, combine the carrots, rutabaga, and water. Bring to a boil. Reduce heat to medium; cover and cook for 13 to 15 minutes.

3. In a small saucepan, combine the remaining ingredients; cook, uncovered, over medium heat for 2 to 3 minutes or until butter is melted.

4. Drain vegetables; add butter mixture. Cook for 3 to 4 minutes or until vegetables are glazed, stirring occasionally.

Chapter 4
Preventing Colorectal Cancer

Colorectal cancer, also called colon cancer or large bowel cancer, is the third most common cancer in the United States. Colon cancer symptoms may include a change in bowel habits or bleeding, but usually colon cancer strikes without symptoms. Understand your risks and how your doctor can identify polyps before your life is at risk. New research seems to come out weekly about what you should or shouldn't be eating, drinking, or doing to prevent it. Learn what you can do to lower your risk.

Colorectal Polyps

Colorectal cancer causes an estimated 55,000 deaths every year and is the second most common cancer killer in the United States. With 138,000 new cases of colorectal cancer diagnosed annually, men and women are equally at risk for this type of cancer.

All colon cancers begin as polyps. Polyps are small, abnormal growths that form on the wall of the colon. If left untreated, polyps may become cancerous over time. However, if polyps are identified and then removed at an early stage, then they do not have the opportunity to become cancerous.

Dangers of Diverticulosis

Diverticulosis affects the large intestine, or colon. Normally, a colon is strong and relatively smooth. When a person has diverticulosis, there are weak spots in the walls. Those weak spots create small pouches in the colon that bulge outward. Imagine an inner tube that pokes through a weak place in a tire. Each pouch is about the size of a large pea.

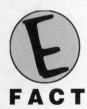

FACT

The disease was first noticed in the United States in the early 1900s. According to the National Digestive Diseases Information Clearinghouse (NDDIC), at about the same time, processed foods were introduced into the American diet. Many processed foods contain refined, low-fiber flour. Unlike whole-wheat flour, refined flour has no wheat bran.

A single pouch in the colon is defined as a diverticulum. Diverticulosis can occur anywhere in the colon, but most are found in the lower left side. That portion is called the sigmoid colon, and it is where the colon is the narrowest and the inner pressure the highest.

Discovering Polyps

As many as 80 percent of the people who have diverticulosis never realize they have it. It is actually a very common disorder in people over age sixty. In fact, more than half of all people between the ages of sixty and eighty have diverticulosis, and nearly everyone over age eighty has the condition.

Diverticulosis can be difficult to diagnose because it usually causes no symptoms. It is usually discovered during an intestinal examination. Tests like barium enema X-ray, flexible sigmoidoscopy, or colonoscopy examinations can all be helpful diagnostic tools.

Diverticulitis Risks

When there are pouches on the colon, it is called diverticulosis. When the pouches become inflamed and/or infected, it is called diverticulitis. The pouches get infected due to the bacteria in the stool that gets lodged in the pouch. Diverticulitis can cause pain and tenderness on the left side of the lower abdomen.

If infection occurs, patients can expect to experience fever, nausea, vomiting, chills, cramping, and constipation. The extent of the infection and complications will affect the severity of symptoms. Diverticulitis can create health difficulties like bleeding, infections, tears, or blockages in the bowel.

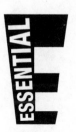

Studies in the *New England Journal of Medicine* have shown that a daily aspirin decreases the number of polyps in patients at high risk for colon polyps, which are precursors to colon cancer. Talk to your physician about including an aspirin in your daily diet.

When you are faced with diverticulitis, you will usually be prescribed antibiotics. When diverticulitis has minor symptoms, oral antibiotics are usually effective. Examples of commonly prescribed antibiotics include ciprofloxacin (Cipro), metronidazole (Flagyl), cephalexin (Keflex), and doxycycline (Vibramycin). Acute diverticulitis attacks will usually require patients to be limited to liquid diets or low-fiber foods. In severe diverticulitis with high fever and pain, some patients will need to be hospitalized and given intravenous antibiotics.

Diverticulosis Causes and Treatment

Constipation appears to be a culprit for the condition. When you are constipated, it makes the muscles strain to move stool that is too hard. That strain is the main cause of increased pressure in the colon. This excess pressure might cause the weak spots in the colon to bulge out. Other risk factors include:

- Diet low in fiber content or high in fat
- High intake of meat and red meat
- Increasing age
- Constipation
- Connective tissue disorders that may cause weakness in the colon wall

Diverticulitis Treatment

Once diverticula have formed, there is no way to reverse the process. The pouches are there for the rest of your life. Some people find that eating nuts and seeds during an attack of diverticulitis can be irritating to the inflamed intestinal lining.

When to Seek Medical Care

Seek medical attention if you have these symptoms:

- Persistent abdominal pain
- Persistent unexplained fevers
- Persistent diarrhea
- Persistent vomiting
- A urinary tract infection that won't go away

Any time you have bleeding from your rectum, you should see your health care provider right away. This is true even if the bleeding stops on its own. Bleeding may be a sign of diverticulitis or other serious diseases. If there is a lot of blood or a steady flow of blood, go to a hospital emergency department immediately.

During diverticulitis attacks, many doctors suggest mild pain medication and bowel rest. Bowel rest usually involves two to three days of clear fluids (no food at all), so your colon may heal without having to work.

Preventing Diverticulitis

Once you have had diverticulitis, your odds are high it will return. To reduce the odds of diverticula becoming inflamed or infected, follow the same recommendations to prevent constipation.

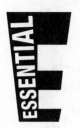

For chronic constipation, try one of these variations of pudding power: In a blender, blend 1 cup crushed 100 percent bran flakes with 1½ cups of canned pears in their own juice. You can substitute the pears with 1 cup applesauce and ½ cup prune juice. To take the pudding, drink an 8-ounce glass of warm water, followed by a tablespoon of pudding power a day for the first week, two tablespoons a day for the second week, and so on, up to five tablespoons a day.

Eat a high-fiber diet, drink plenty of fluids, and exercise regularly. Aim for 38 grams of fiber per day for men and 25 grams per day for women.

Colon Cancer

Cancer that begins in the colon is called colon cancer, and cancer that begins in the rectum is called rectal cancer. Cancers affecting either of these organs may also be called colorectal cancer. Colorectal cancer is cancer of the colon and rectum, two parts of the digestive system also known as the large intestine.

Risk Factors for Colorectal Cancer

There are several risk factors for developing colorectal cancer. Having one or more of these risk factors does not guarantee that a person will develop colorectal cancer; it just increases the chances. While you cannot change your past medical history, your genetics, or your age, you can impact your future medical history. Getting appropriate screenings and developing a healthy lifestyle can increase your odds of staying healthy longer.

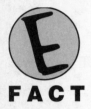

Don't let the price of testing keep you from getting the care you need. Medicare covers colorectal cancer screening and will pay part or all of the cost of a fecal occult blood test, flexible sigmoidoscopy, barium enema, or colonoscopy. If fees are a concern, then talk to your doctor or local hospital about possible sliding-scale fees based on your income.

Women are just as likely as men to develop colorectal cancer, but age is a risk factor. The older you get, the more likely you are to develop colorectal cancer. Once you hit forty years old, your chances of developing cancer increase, but especially so after the age of fifty. In some cases it can occur in teenagers and in other young adults.

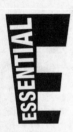

For some people, seeking the advice of a genetic counselor may be worthwhile. Medical researchers have learned that changes in specific genes may well raise the risk of colorectal cancer. If there are several cases of colorectal cancer in your family, you may find it helpful to talk with a genetic counselor.

Medical researchers propose that your diet may place you at a higher risk for colorectal cancer. Diets that are high in fat and calories and low in fiber may pose a higher risk. In addition, your family genetics may play a role in how likely you are to develop colorectal cancer. If you are a close relative of someone who has had colorectal cancer or another chronic digestive condition, you may have a higher-than-average risk of developing colorectal cancer.

Your own medical story impacts your likelihood of getting colorectal cancer. Women who have a history of cancer in the ovary, uterus, or breast may have a slightly higher chance of developing colorectal cancer. If a person has already had colorectal cancer, then they are at a higher risk of developing colorectal disease a second time.

Symptoms of Colorectal Cancer

Many cases of colorectal cancer have no symptoms. That's why annual screening is so important. However, if you have these symptoms and either have not yet been tested or it has been longer than a year since you were tested, then contact your physician:

- Frequent gas pains
- Blood in or on the stool
- Diarrhea or constipation
- A feeling that the bowel has not emptied completely
- Blood in the stool or rectal bleeding
- Persistent change in bowel habits
- Change in the shape of the stool (such as pencil-thin feces, or presence of black, tar-like stool)
- Pain in the abdomen or rectum
- Cramping
- A frequent feeling of fullness in the rectum
- Frequent false urges to defecate
- Persistent or alternating bouts of constipation or diarrhea
- Weakness and fatigue
- Weight loss and loss of appetite
- Soilage
- Protrusion from the anal opening
- Ulcer near the anus

Screening for Colorectal Cancer

According to the American Cancer Society, colorectal cancer is one of the leading causes of cancer-related deaths in the United States. The good news is that early diagnosis often leads to a complete cure. With proper screening, colon cancer can be detected before symptoms develop, when it is most curable. People over fifty should be screened for colorectal cancer by their physician. Several tests are recommended to screen for colon cancer:

- An annual fecal occult blood test, which checks for minute traces of blood in the stool.
- A flexible colonoscopy once every five to seven years to detect colorectal cancer at its earliest and most treatable stage.
- If, for some reason, a colonoscopy cannot be performed, then a double contrast barium enema (DCBE), a series of X-rays of the colon and rectum, is a reasonable second choice. The patient is given an enema with a solution that contains barium, which outlines the colon and rectum on the X-rays.
- A digital rectal exam (DRE) is an annual exam in which the doctor inserts a lubricated, gloved finger into the rectum to feel for abnormal areas.
- A colonoscopy, performed as often as your physician suggests, is recommended for high-risk patients of any age with prior history of cancer, a strong family history of the disease, or a predisposing chronic digestive condition such as inflammatory bowel disease.

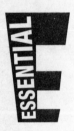

Colorectal cancer screening costs range from $1,400 to $3,000, and more than half of Americans do not have guaranteed health insurance coverage for them. You can help advocate for better coverage by going to *http://coveryourbutt.org*.

Take Control of Your Colon Health

You have a great deal of power when it comes to improving your health. Maintain a healthy weight, talk to a genetic counselor, don't smoke, and exercise. Even reducing your radiation exposure can be one more step toward protecting your colon.

Listen to Your Body

You aren't supposed to hurt. Digestive problems are not normal. Don't brush off uncomfortable signals your body is trying to give you. If something doesn't feel right, get it checked out.

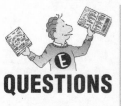

Is it okay to eat red meat if I'm concerned about colon cancer?
Go for the fish instead. In a major study of 478,000 people, those who ate six ounces of red and/or processed meat daily were one-third more likely to have colon cancer than those who ate less than one ounce per day.

Regular Checkups

The facts are simple. You could have colon cancer or a precancerous condition and not know it. While researchers believe diet, exercise, genetics, and lifestyle all play a role in your colon health, even people who do all the right things get cancer. If you avoid getting tests and exams done on a regular basis, you are taking a risk with your health.

Eating for Colon Health

You cannot prevent cancer by eating certain things, but scientists do believe what you choose to eat (and avoid) can decrease your likelihood of developing cancer. The following recipes were developed using the latest in colorectal research and are all low in fat and high in fiber.

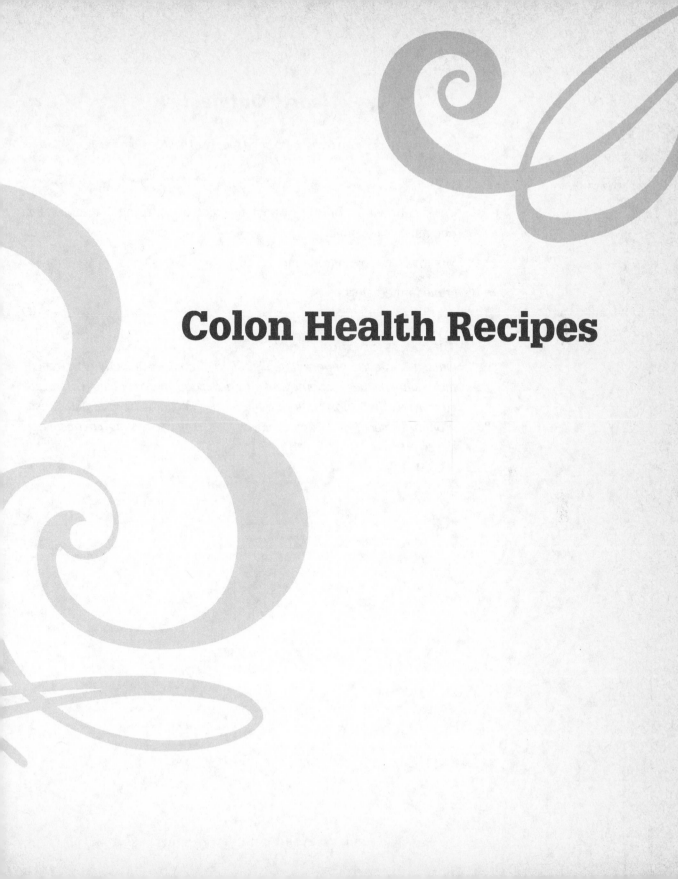

Colon Health Recipes

Hearty Oatmeal

Serves 1

Ingredients

1 cup instant oatmeal, uncooked

1¾ cups water, rice milk, or soy milk

2 tablespoons ground flaxseed

2 tablespoons chopped walnuts

2 tablespoons maple syrup

2 tablespoons raisins

Walnuts and flaxseed are both good sources of healthful omega-3s.

1. Cook oatmeal according to package directions, using 1¾ cup water, rice milk, or soy milk.

2. Mix in remaining ingredients.

3. Serve immediately.

Omega-3s for Colon Health

Omega-3s are too important to skip! In a fourteen-year study of 320 men, those who ate the most omega-3 fatty acids had 76 percent less colorectal cancer risk than those who ate the least. Omega-3s from walnuts, fish, ground flaxseed, and canola oil may cut cancer-boosting chemicals in the colon.

Lemon Artichoke Chicken

Artichokes are high in magnesium. Eating lots of dairy, fruits, vegetables, grains, and nuts—all high in magnesium—cut the number of tumors caused by colon cancer by 34 percent and rectal cancer by 55 percent in a Swedish study.

1. Preheat the oven to 350°F.

2. Heat olive oil in a large skillet over medium heat. Add the onion and cook, stir until it is soft and translucent, about 5 minutes. Add the garlic, artichokes, mushrooms, lemon juice, and peppers, cook for 2 more minutes and set aside.

3. Slice the chicken breasts into ½"-wide strips. Season the chicken pieces with rosemary, salt, and pepper and lay in a large baking dish.

4. Spoon the artichoke mixture evenly over the chicken and add the wine and broth.

5. Bake for 20 minutes, until you can pierce the chicken and get clear juices.

Serves 4

Ingredients
1 tablespoon olive oil
1 small onion, diced
1 tablespoon minced garlic
1 (9-ounce) bag frozen
    artichoke hearts,
    quartered
1 cup sliced mushrooms
1 teaspoon lemon juice
1 red pepper, seeded and
    sliced into strips
4 skinless, boneless chicken
    breasts
1 teaspoon chopped, fresh
    rosemary or thyme
Salt and pepper to taste
¼ cup dry sherry or white
    wine
1 cup low-sodium chicken
    broth

Kiwi Banana Smoothie

Serves 2

Ingredients

2 kiwi fruit, peeled and sliced
1 ripe banana, peeled
¼ cup plain low-fat yogurt
3 ice cubes
1 teaspoon vanilla
½ teaspoon nutmeg

High daily levels of vitamin B6 may reduce the risk of getting colon cancer by 58 percent, claims a study from Harvard Medical School. Reductions in cancer risk started showing up at levels of just 3.3 milligrams a day. Bananas and kiwi are both good sources of B6.

1. Place the kiwi, banana, yogurt, and ice cubes in a blender.

2. Process until smooth, adding vanilla and nutmeg to taste.

3. Divide into 2 glasses.

Turkey and Avocado Open-Faced Sandwich

Serves 2

Ingredients

½ avocado
1 tablespoon lemon juice
2 slices rye bread
6 slices hormone- and
    antibiotic-free turkey

In a Finnish study, those who ate about 4½ slices of whole-grain rye bread every day for 4 weeks had reduced levels of bile acids thought to promote colon cancer by an average of 26 percent. Look for "whole rye flour" or "whole rye meal" on the label.

1. Mash the avocado with a tablespoon of lemon juice.

2. Spoon over a slice of rye bread and top with the sliced turkey.

Orange Nut Salad

A Harvard University study showed that women who took in 400 micrograms of folate (the food form of folic acid) each day cut their risk of colon cancer by 40 percent. Folate can be found in beans, leafy greens, and orange juice.

1. Combine orange juice, lemon juice, honey, mustard, orange rind, and salt in small bowl.

2. Whisk in oil until well blended. Refrigerate until ready to use.

3. Wash and dry the romaine lettuce on paper towels or in a salad spinner. Tear into bite size pieces and place in a large salad bowl.

4. Combine the remainder of the salad ingredients.

5. Pour dressing over salad immediately before serving.

Serves 4

Ingredients

Dressing:
3 tablespoons orange juice
1 tablespoon lemon juice
1 tablespoon honey
2 teaspoons Dijon-style mustard
2 teaspoons orange rind, grated
½ teaspoon salt
⅔ cup vegetable oil

Salad:
1 head romaine lettuce
3 tablespoons red onion, chopped
1 cup mandarin oranges
1 tablespoon fresh parsley, minced
½ cup pecans

Savory Cabbage Soup

Serves 4

Ingredients
1 head cabbage
6 green onions
2 green peppers
1 can diced tomatoes
1 bunch celery
2 carrots
3 cups cooked cannellini
    beans
2 cans low-sodium vegetable
    broth
½ to 1 teaspoon dried dill
    weed
1 soup can of water
Salt and pepper to taste

Eat cruciferous vegetables. Cabbage, broccoli, Brussels sprouts, and cauliflower have anti-carcinogens, but be wary if they give you indigestion.

1. Cut the vegetables into bite-sized pieces and shred cabbage.

2. Sauté the cabbage, onions, green peppers, tomatoes, celery, and carrots 3 to 5 minutes in a nonstick frying pan.

3. Add vegetables and other ingredients in a medium stockpot. Add water to just cover the mixture.

4. Bring to a boil, then lower heat to simmer until vegetables are soft. Add salt and pepper to taste.

Grilled Asparagus

Serves 4

Ingredients
1 bunch asparagus
2 tablespoons olive oil
1 teaspoon lemon juice
1 teaspoon lemon zest
Salt and pepper to taste

Lutein is a carotenoid and antioxidant found in green, leafy vegetables, bell peppers, asparagus, tomatoes, and corn. Along with other antioxidants (vitamins A, C and E, and selenium), lutein has been shown to reduce the risk of colorectal cancer.

1. Trim bottoms of asparagus.

2. Lightly brush with olive oil.

3. Grill over medium heat or under broiler for 3 minutes.

4. Sprinkle with lemon juice, then lemon zest. Add salt and pepper as desired.

Chickpea Salad

Chickpeas contain calcium, which may help prevent colon cancer. Women who consumed at least 800 mg of calcium daily had 25 percent less colorectal cancer risk than those who got no more than 400 mg, according to an 8½-year study at the University of Minnesota.

1. Combine the chickpeas, garlic, olive oil, lemon juice, parsley, and anchovy in a large bowl.

2. Season with salt and pepper. Taste, and adjust seasoning as necessary.

3. Chill, covered, until ready to serve.

4. When ready to serve, toss with baby spinach and tomatoes. Add parmesan cheese as desired on top.

Serves 2

Ingredients
1 can (14-ounce) chickpeas, drained
1 garlic clove, crushed
1 tablespoon olive oil
Juice of ½ lemon
Handful chopped parsley
½ anchovy
Salt and pepper to taste
2 large handfuls baby spinach
1 cup cherry tomatoes
Shaved parmesan cheese for garnish

Tofu Stir-Fry

A good source of protein, B-vitamins, and iron, tofu is a perfect replacement for red meat in your diet. In recipes, tofu acts like a sponge and has the miraculous ability to soak up any flavor that is added to it. Cubes of firm tofu can be added to any casserole or soup.

1. Drain and cut tofu into 1" cubes. Wash, trim, and cut vegetables into bite-sized pieces.

2. Sauté the garlic, onion, ginger, carrot, and broccoli in sesame oil, lemon juice, and olive oil about 5 minutes.

3. Add peppers and tofu, sauté 3 minutes.

4. Add teriyaki sauce, snow peas, and bean sprouts. Stir, cover, and simmer for 1 minute. Serve with rice or noodles.

Serves 4

Ingredients
1 (12-ounce) package light firm tofu
3 cups vegetables (broccoli, carrots, bell pepper, snowpeas)
1 teaspoon minced fresh garlic
3 whole green onions, finely chopped
2 tablespoons fresh ginger, grated, including peel
¼ teaspoon hot sesame oil
2 tablespoons fresh-squeezed lemon juice
½ teaspoon extra-virgin olive oil
2 tablespoons light teriyaki sauce or tamari sauce
1 cup bean sprouts

Garlic Greens with White Beans

Eating garlic regularly may reduce the risk of esophageal, colon, and stomach cancer. Researchers suggest it may be due to garlic's ability to reduce the formation of carcinogenic compounds.

Serves 4

Ingredients

1 large bunch greens (spinach, mustard greens, kale, or broccoli rabe), about 10 cups

4 tablespoons plus 1 teaspoon extra-virgin olive oil

3 minced garlic cloves

1 teaspoon dry white wine

1 teaspoon lemon juice

¼ teaspoon sea salt

1 cup (or more) vegetable broth or low-salt chicken broth

1 (15-ounce) can white beans, rinsed, drained

1 teaspoon vinegar

1. Wash greens, remove stems, and cut into 1" strips.

2. Heat 4 tablespoons oil in large nonstick skillet over medium heat. Add garlic, white wine, lemon juice, and sea salt, and stir for 1 minute, until garlic is golden.

3. Using tongs, add greens a cup at a time to skillet and stir just until beginning to wilt before adding more.

4. Slowly add broth, cover, and simmer until greens are tender, about 5 to 10 minutes.

5. Add beans then simmer uncovered until liquid is almost absorbed and beans are heated, about 3 minutes.

6. Drizzle with 1 teaspoon each of vinegar and oil.

Chapter 5
Food Intolerance and Allergies

Some people can become either acutely ill or suffer a variety of seemingly unrelated symptoms caused by certain foods they are eating. A food intolerance is your body's way of saying that this food is not right for your body. The incidence of food intolerances has increased five times over the past two decades. Food intolerances can cause symptoms ranging from nausea, bloating, abdominal pain, and diarrhea to joint pain, asthma, skin rashes, and fatigue. You may have a food intolerance and not realize it.

What's the Difference?

The symptoms of food allergy and food sensitivity are very similar, but have completely different causes. If you have a true food allergy, your body reacts quickly and dramatically, using the same system it would if you had hay fever and inhaled a lot of pollen all at once. In response to your eating the offending food, certain cells release the chemical histamine, which can cause you to start sneezing, wheezing, or break out in hives.

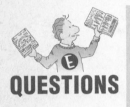

QUESTIONS

What is one of the main differences between a food allergy and a food sensitivity?
One of the easiest ways to tell the difference is in the amount of time it takes to display symptoms. A true allergy shows symptoms very quickly, while a food sensitivity may take a few hours to present.

The mechanism behind a food sensitivity is completely different and does not involve histamine release. With a sensitivity, hours after eating the culprit food, and after it is partially digested, large, incompletely digested molecules "leak" through your intestinal wall. These "mega-molecules" latch on to specific antibodies (termed *antigen-antibody complexes*), travel through your bloodstream, and attach themselves in certain vulnerable areas (joints, bronchial tubes, skin). The treatment of food sensitivities combines avoidance of the offending foods and repair of the "leaky gut" lining.

Lactose intolerance generally develops in middle age and runs in families and certain ethnic groups. Since humans really only need milk products when they are children, it is not surprising that the ability to digest this particular food group would lessen as people grow older.

Gluten intolerance (celiac disease) is not an allergy nor does it involve an enzyme. Rather, for reasons unknown, gluten itself becomes toxic to the delicate cells of the small intestine and virtually destroys them, impairing their ability to absorb food. The only treatment for this illness is total avoidance of gluten.

Causes

No one knows why some people are allergic or sensitive to some foods, but not others. Some allergies, like peanut allergies, are more likely to run in families, so there is some genetic component. Stress has been shown to play a role in allergic reactions. You may show an allergic response to a food for a period of time—even years—but it can disappear for random periods of time. Reactions may reappear when some other stress is present.

As opposed to true food allergies, people develop food sensitivities when they eat the same food day in and day out.

For example, after learning they have developed wheat sensitivity, some people realize they have been eating and snacking on one wheat product or another three or four times a day for years. It's really not known why some people develop gluten sensitivity.

Common Food Offenders

Some food offenders can be difficult to identify because the food "trigger" may be found in a wide variety of products. Corn, for example, can appear not only in corn flakes, or canned corn, but might also sweeten a wheat-based breakfast cereal with high-fructose corn syrup. You may become sensitive to preservatives and additives found in processed and packaged food. For example, inulin is an additive made of fruit residues that can be found in butter, ice cream, yogurt, cereals and jams.

Other common food triggers include:

- Artificial additives (MSG, coloring, and so on)
- Artificial sweeteners
- Citrus (mostly oranges)
- Coffee and caffeine
- Corn and corn derivatives
- Dairy products
- Eggs
- Peanuts
- Shellfish
- Soy
- Wheat and refined flour

Symptoms

Symptoms commonly associated with food intolerances include, but are not limited to, digestive symptoms such as nausea, gas, bloating, diarrhea, abdominal pain, and other gastrointestinal symptoms. Nondigestive symptoms include fatigue, brain "fog," sinus congestion, asthma, joint and muscle pain, skin rashes, and a general feeling of chronic ill health.

Food Allergy Treatments

If you are having a mild food allergy reaction with facial swelling and hives, taking an over-the-counter antihistamine may be helpful to relieve your symptoms. There is no magic pill that can let you eat peanut butter or shellfish if you are prone to having a severe reaction. If, however, you are experiencing wheezing or shortness of breath, you should immediately go to an emergency room for treatment. The major risk for severe allergies is the potential of going into life-threatening anaphylactic shock. You may also wish to wear some type of medical alert bracelet in case of a severe allergy reaction.

ALERT!

If you or someone in your family has a severe food allergy, you may want to consider purchasing Food Allergy Restaurant Cards to share at restaurants you frequent, which explain the food allergy, warns about cross-contamination, lists potentially dangerous foods and ingredients, and tells when to call 911.

How to Check for Food Intolerances

With true food allergies, with sudden onset of face and lip swelling, general "itchiness," and skin rash, it's generally easy to identify the offending food because the reaction occurs so quickly. Because the symptoms of food sensitivities may occur one or two days after eating the offending food, these are much harder to diagnose. Screening blood tests, which check for up to

100 commonly eaten foods, can be helpful, but the most valuable diagnostic tool is a food sensitivity elimination diet. Your doctor can order food sensitivity blood tests, as well as tests to check for lactose intolerance and gluten sensitivity.

Whether you opt for blood tests, skin tests, or elimination diets, you can begin to identify the culprits in your diet causing you grief. Very few skin tests work for food sensitivities, but you may find that a combination of dietary changes and diagnostic tests give you the answers you're craving.

Elimination Diet

There are several different methods of trying an elimination diet to identify problematic foods. Regardless of what you try, keep an accurate food journal for the time period you are testing. Do not try to rely on your memory to track what you ate when, and what symptoms you had for how long.

The easiest elimination diet involves you completely eliminating all dairy, egg, corn, wheat, citrus, and soy products for at least one week. Since these are by far the most common offenders, if, after one week of complete elimination, you feel exactly the same, with absolutely no improvement of your symptoms, then food intolerances are probably not present. However, if you feel "better," you may be on to something. Now it's time to play detective. Add one food group back into your diet every three days and record your physical response. If nothing occurs, remain on that food, and add the next on the list. Ultimately, you'll likely unearth the guilty party. If you feel better eliminating wheat, be sure to have your doctor test you for gluten sensitivity (celiac disease).

Diagnostic Testing

The majority of problematic food sensitivities are the delayed-onset type (IgG), taking hours to days to occur. Immediate reactions are easier to identify and eliminate because they have a fast onset (IgE antibody). (Skin prick testing identifies only IgE type, and is better for environmental sensitivities.) The blood testing screens multiple foods for reactions based on both immediate and delayed onset (IgG and IgE antibody reactions).

Dairy Intolerance

Three out of every four people over age forty-five can no longer digest milk protein (termed *lactose intolerance*). True dairy allergy often occurs in infants, but is usually outgrown by the time they are two or three years old. Rashes, hives, vomiting, or diarrhea are the most likely symptoms. Casein, a protein in the milk, is what creates problems; it's not the milk sugar (lactose).

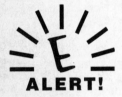

When looking for milk substitutes, pay attention if you are allergic to gluten. Many rice milks contain gluten. Some products have this clearly labeled, while some don't include the information or keep it hidden.

Casein can be difficult to avoid, particularly since many "dairy-free" products (whipped toppings, creamers, and so on) contain casein. It may be helpful to watch for the "kosher" symbol on foods, making sure it is not followed by a "D," which indicates the presence of dairy.

Meet Calcium Requirements

The daily recommended intake of calcium varies according to age, but will average between 500 mg and 1,000 mg according to the National Academy of Science. Starting the day with a bowl of one of the fortified cereals will give you as much as 1,000 mg of calcium.

Lactose Intolerance

There is a perception that lactose intolerance is a disease. It isn't—it is just when a person's body cannot digest and metabolize lactose, a carbohydrate. Lactose, also known as milk sugar, is found in dairy products, which are, of course, made from the milk of animals.

Lactose intolerance may be primary, lasting all of a person's life, or secondary. Secondary lactose intolerance may develop after a patient's intestinal lining has been injured by allergy or infection. This type of lactose intolerance will last only until the intestinal lining is healed. Because it is very common in children after experiencing a diarrhea-producing viral illness, many health care providers recommend delaying the introduction of milk while the child is still recovering.

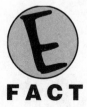

Dose dependence means some people will sometimes not have side effects to a certain medication or substance until they eat more than a certain amount. The side effects are "dependent" on the dose. This is especially true for many people who can't stomach lactose. They might be able to have ¼ cup of milk on their cereal and not have problems but will experience symptoms if they drink a full glass of milk.

Symptoms of lactose intolerance include:

- Abdominal bloating
- Gas
- Stomach cramps
- Flatulence
- Diarrhea
- Bad breath (generally much worse than typical morning breath and resistant to good oral hygiene)

Milk Strategies

Lactose intolerance may be inconvenient, but it is fairly easily managed. You do, however, need to be proactive and try several different strategies for getting milk's nutritional benefits in your diet. Once you have identified lactose as a problem for you, carefully avoid any lactose-containing dairy products for several weeks. Gradually, increase the amount of lactose you eat, beginning with just a tablespoon of milk. Every couple of days, double the amount you take in until you reach your tolerance.

It may be that you can drink milk, but you need to do so in smaller but more frequent servings. While more expensive, you may prefer to switch to reduced-lactose milk, such as Lactaid. You can also take a lactase capsule when you are going to consume dairy products.

Reading labels is very important when it comes to avoiding lactose. In fact, a product may even be labeled lactose free but still contain sodium caseinate or casein, a milk protein, which may give you problems. Common offenders include soy or rice cheese alternatives and sour cream alternatives.

Treatment

Lactose enzyme capsules work for many people. By taking a pill containing the lactase with your meal that contains lactose, it's easier to tolerate the lactose in some foods. Fermented milk products such as yogurt, containing *L. bulgaricus* and *S. thermophilus*, may help decrease the symptoms of lactose intolerance and seem to be tolerated fairly well by most people who are lactose intolerant.

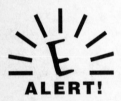

Grocery items that may contain lactose include processed and prepared foods such as bread, baked goods, candy, cookies, breakfast drinks, chocolate drink mixes, sauces and gravies, frosting, frozen dinners, pancake and biscuit mixes, coffee creamer, and snack foods.

Lactose-Free Diet

Eating a well-rounded diet is important for everybody—regardless of food sensitivities. People who are eating a lactose-free diet need to be aware that their eating plan can create some nutritional deficiencies, especially calcium. If you are eating a lactose-free diet, be intentional when shopping and look for foods rich in calcium and vitamin D. For example, bread and orange juice are now available in calcium-enriched versions. Usually, you can make substitutions in recipes measure for measure (1 cup soy milk for 1 cup regular milk, 1 ounce soy cream cheese for 1 ounce regular cream cheese). The calcium in soy milk is not as easily absorbed as cow's milk.

Gluten Sensitivities

Gluten, a protein found in wheat, rye, oats, and barley and their derivatives, causes celiac disease. Sufferers of celiac disease experience changes in their small intestine and often a loss of their ability to absorb crucial nutrients. Up to 1 million Americans are intolerant to gluten.

Celiac Disease

Celiac disease is a digestive disorder that is triggered by eating the protein gluten, which is found in the grains wheat, rye, and barley. There is no cure for the disease, but it can be controlled through strict avoidance of foods that contain gluten. Many people with celiac disease remain undiagnosed, since the symptoms are often similar to other conditions. Physicians often misdiagnose celiacs as having illnesses such as irritable bowel syndrome, food allergies, chronic fatigue, anorexia, or malnutrition.

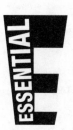

Probiotics have been shown to reduce the toxicity of gluten. Studies have shown a benefit of probiotic bacteria that are added to gluten-containing breads. They may be especially beneficial in those with celiac disease, potentially protecting against cross-contamination exposure.

Other Illnesses Affected by Gluten

People with many other conditions can also benefit from a gluten-free diet, including ADD, multiple sclerosis, lactose intolerance (up to 48 percent of people with celiac are also lactose intolerant), autism, chronic fatigue, indigestion, and malnutrition.

Buying Gluten-Free Products

People who need to eat a gluten-free diet may eat rice, corn, potatoes, all kinds of vegetables and fruit, eggs, cheese, milk, meat and fish, nuts, seeds, and beans. Read product labels carefully to ensure the products are not cooked with wheat flour, batter, breadcrumbs, or sauces.

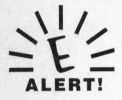

Research shows celiac disease progresses faster in men, depleting more nutrients and damaging bones. Dr. Alessio Fasano, medical director at the University of Maryland's Center for Celiac Research, says celiac disease is a leading cause of male osteoporosis.

What makes eating a gluten-free diet tricky is that there is a long list of forbidden ingredients (e.g., dextrin and malto-dextrin, citric acid), which are often snuck into processed foods. As a simple rule, processed and prepared food is off limits unless it is marked gluten-free. However, there is no federal regulation that defines the term "gluten-free" used in the labeling of foods.

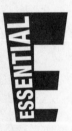

The Essential Gluten-Free Grocery Guide is a full-color publication designed to help you find gluten-free foods. From brand-name ice cream to private-label canned soup, this product guide covers more than 20,000 gluten-free foods found in popular grocery stores. Find it at *www .triumphdining.com.*

Other products with gluten include:

- Lip stick/lip balm (use Burt's Bees beeswax lip balm)
- Sunscreen (use Banana Boat children's sunscreen)
- Children's stickers and price tags
- Stamps and envelopes
- Washing machine detergent (use Arm & Hammer baking soda detergent)
- Soaps and shampoos
- Toothpaste and mouthwash (use Tom's of Maine toothpaste)
- Cosmetics

Gluten can be hidden in caramel coloring, modified food starch, and "flavor enhancers." Check labels before you buy.

Eating Out Gluten Free

Restaurants that advertise organic foods are more likely to accommodate food allergies. Check out a restaurant online first. Many chain restaurants offer gluten-free menus, but you'll have to ask to get it. Call ahead if you're not sure. The best time to reach a restaurant is about 2 P.M.—between the lunch and dinner rush.

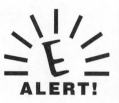

Information and communication are crucial for celiac patients when it comes to eating out, purchasing foods, or even taking medications, because something as simple and small as a tiny piece of crouton can cause hours of suffering. Diane Craig, chairwoman of the Sacramento Celiac Sprue Association, says while many people have heard of the disease, misconceptions remain about what celiac patients can eat—including the idea that just a little gluten won't hurt.

Any Thai restaurant without Chinese or Japanese food on the menu will likely accommodate you easily. Oaxacan food (Mexican food from the region of Oaxaca) is often made from scratch. As with any restaurant that serves sauces and salsas, ask if flour is used in the sauce/salsa/mole. Also ask if the oil for chips is also used to fry foods that contain flour.

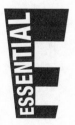

Check out *www.CeliacChicks.com*—a great website that bills itself as the cool guide to a hip and healthy celiac lifestyle. It offers great tips, restaurant suggestions, and a list of gluten-free bloggers.

Lactose- and Gluten-Free Recipes

Banana Delight Dessert (Lactose-Free)

Serves 2

Ingredients
2 ripe bananas
1 tablespoon maple syrup
1 tablespoon cocoa powder
2 teaspoons vanilla
¼ teaspoon nutmeg
¼ teaspoon cinnamon

Buy raw cocoa powder rather then cocoa powder treated with alkali (also called Dutch cocoa) because that alkali destroys a lot of good antioxidants, which are naturally present in cocoa.

1. Blend all ingredients together, then place in freezer.

2. Freeze and serve.

Rich Broccoli Soup (Lactose-Free)

Serves 4

Ingredients
1 (16-ounce) bag of frozen
    chopped broccoli
3 medium red potatoes,
    peeled and chopped
1 small onion, diced
1 teaspoon lemon juice
1 teaspoon Italian seasoning
½ teaspoon salt
⅛ teaspoon freshly ground
    black pepper
3 cups vegetable broth
1 cup soy or rice milk

You don't have to avoid creamy soup if you can't have dairy. Blending makes this soup rich and creamy.

1. In saucepan, add broccoli, potatoes, onion, lemon juice, and seasonings to broth.

2. Heat to boiling and simmer for 30 minutes or until potatoes are tender.

3. In a blender, combine ingredients of saucepan with milk. Blend until smooth then serve.

Tahini (Gluten-free and Lactose-Free)

Tahini is a simple paste made from crushed sesame seeds. It is versatile and high in calcium, with 2 tablespoons offering 130mg of calcium.

Yields 4 cups

Ingredients
5 cups sesame seeds
1½ cups peanut oil

1. Preheat oven to 350°F.

2. Toast sesame seeds on a baking sheet for 5 to 10 minutes. Frequently turn the seeds with a spatula and do not allow to brown. They should be golden.

3. Cool for 20 minutes.

4. Pour sesame seeds into food processor and add oil. Blend for 2 minutes.

5. Process until it is very smooth. The goal is a thick, yet pourable texture. Add more oil and blend until desired consistency. Serve with pitas.

Dairy-Free Dip (Lactose-Free)

This is the perfect dip for fruit, or to serve with angel food cake.

Serves 4

Ingredients
½ cup nondairy imitation
  cream cheese
½ cup nondairy imitation
  sour cream
1 tablespoon lime or lemon
  juice
1 tablespoon honey
1 tablespoon seedless
  raspberry jam

1. Combine cream cheese and sour cream until smooth.

2. Add lime juice, honey, and jam.

3. Mix well and serve.

Gluten-Free Corn Casserole

Serves 6

Ingredients

8 ounces crumbled corn bread (made without wheat flour)
1 cup lactose-free milk
Small piece green bell pepper (if tolerated)
¼ small onion (if tolerated)
2 eggs
¾ teaspoon salt
⅛ teaspoon pepper
2 tablespoons butter or margarine
1½ cups cooked or canned whole kernel corn, drained

This is perfect for potluck lunches and no one will know it's made to accommodate food sensitivities.

1. Preheat oven to 350°F and grease a 1-quart casserole.

2. Put all remaining ingredients except corn in blender, cover, chop, and pour over soft crumbs. Mix together.

3. Add corn to casserole; mix well.

4. Bake about 1 hour or until a knife inserted in center comes out clean.

Salmon Wraps (Lactose-Free)

Serves 4

Ingredients

2 cans or pouches (6 to 7.1 ounces each) skinless, boneless salmon, drained and chunked
8 wedges spreadable light Swiss cheese
2 tablespoons fresh chives, chopped
1 tablespoon lemon juice
1 tablespoon chopped dill
4 large (10") whole-wheat flour tortillas
4 cups chopped or thinly sliced assorted fresh vegetables

Vegetables can include cucumber, spinach, bean sprouts, shredded carrots, broccoli, and/or cabbage.

1. In a medium bowl, blend salmon, Swiss cheese, chives, lemon juice, and dill.

2. Spread salmon–Swiss cheese mixture on each tortilla.

3. Add 1 cup of vegetables to each tortilla and roll up.

Tofu and Chinese Cabbage Soup (Gluten-Free and Lactose-Free)

If you dislike cabbage because of its strong flavor, try it in soup instead. The flavor is much more mellow, but still has crunch.

1. Sauté cabbage and green onions in sesame oil.

2. Add other ingredients, except the snow peas and tofu.

3. Bring to a boil, then simmer on low heat for 10 minutes.

4. Add in snow peas and tofu. Heat for additional 30 minutes or until tofu is heated through.

Serves 4

Ingredients
2 cups firmly packed Chinese cabbage, chopped
¾ cup thinly sliced green onion
1 tablespoon light sesame oil
1 (6-ounce) can sliced water chestnuts, undrained
1 (32-ounce) carton low-sodium vegetable or fat-free gluten-free chicken broth
2 tablespoons dry sherry or wine
2 teaspoons reduced-sodium soy sauce
1 cup snow peas, trimmed and halved
8 ounces soft or firm tofu, cut into ½" cubes

Rice Milk (Gluten-Free and Lactose-Free)

It takes a little extra effort to make your own, but you can cut down on the amount of sugar typically found in commercial rice milk.

1. Place all ingredients in a blender until smooth.

2. Strain twice to be sure to get out any little rice pieces.

3. You can also add almonds before blending or any other calcium supplement.

Serves 4

Ingredients
4 cups hot/warm water
1 cup cooked rice (white or brown)
1 teaspoon vanilla
Gluten-free brown rice syrup to taste

Watermelon Granita
(Gluten-Free and Lactose-Free)

Serves 2

___

Ingredients

4 cups seedless watermelon
    chunks
½ cup sugar
Juice of 1 lemon

*A sweet and satisfying summer treat, you won't miss the
extra sugar in regular sorbet.*

1. In a food processor, purée all the ingredients until smooth.

2. Pour into a shallow, wide pan and freeze for 1 hour.

3. Rake with a fork, then freeze for an additional hour. Repeat.

4. Remove from the freezer, rake, and serve in cups.

Easy Lactose-Free Ice Cream

Serves 1

___

Ingredients

1 package vanilla instant
    breakfast (any flavor will
    work)
1 cup lactose-free milk

It's not the same as ice cream, but it's a pretty good substitute.

1. Mix the instant breakfast and milk as directed, then pour into a cup.

2. Place in freezer until frozen. Eat as is with a spoon, or put in blender for
   a slushier consistency.

Baking Powder (Gluten-Free)

1½ teaspoons of this mixture equals 1 teaspoon of regular baking powder.

Mix well. Store in an airtight container.

Yields 1 cup

Ingredients
⅓ cup baking soda
⅔ cup cream of tartar
⅔ cup Arrowroot (or potato
    starch)

Spinach and Avocado Salad (Gluten-Free and Lactose-Free)

Shellfish allergies can cause severe reactions in individuals that are intolerant to the proteins in fish products, so make sure shrimp is safe for you.

1. Chop tomatoes into halves or quarters.

2. Seed the avocado, scrape out the flesh into a small bowl, and mash it thoroughly with lemon juice.

3. Arrange spinach on a large plate, top with tomatoes, then shrimp, and avocado dressing.

Serves 1

Ingredients
1 cup cherry tomatoes
1 small avocado
3 tablespoons lemon juice
2 cups shredded spinach
⅓ pound cooked salad
    shrimp

Gluten- and Dairy-Free Cake

Serves 10

Ingredients
2 cups white rice flour
1 cup sorhgum flour
2 cups sugar
1 cup casein-free cocoa
   powder
1 teaspoon salt
2 teaspoons baking soda
2 teaspoons xanthan gum or
   guar gum
1 cup cooking oil
1 cup rice milk
1 cup hot water
2 eggs
4 teaspoons vanilla

Instead of the 8" × 8" pans called for in this recipe, you could also pour the batter into a 9" × 13" pan for a larger cake, or use it to make 24 cupcakes.

1. Preheat oven to 350°F, and grease and flour two 8"× 8" pans.

2. Stir all ingredients until well mixed.

3. Pour batter into pans.

4. Bake in oven for 30 minutes.

Pizza Crust (Gluten-Free)

Serves 6

Ingredients
½ teaspoon sugar
1 cup warm water (105°F to
   110°F)
1½ teaspoons dry, active
   yeast
⅔ cup white rice flour
⅓ cup potato starch
1 tablespoon potato flour
1½ teaspoons melted
   vegetable shortening
½ teaspoon salt

The texture is slightly different from traditional pizza crusts, but it has a great flavor.

1. Preheat oven to 425°F. Grease a pizza pan and set aside.

2. In a medium mixing bowl, mix sugar and water, then dissolve the yeast in ½ cup of the warm water. Let set until yeast bubbles and the quantity doubles—about 10 minutes.

3. Add all the rest of the ingredients, using enough of the remaining water to get a soft dough. It should be thick enough to pick up and knead, but feel very soft.

4. Pour dough on pizza pan and spread with a spatula. Leave more at edges for raised sides. Add sauce and toppings of your liking.

5. Bake for 25 to 30 minutes.

Peanut Butter Cookies
(Gluten-Free and Lactose-Free)

If you can't find xanthan gum in your grocery store, you can order it online.

1. Preheat oven to 325°F.

2. Spray a cookie sheets with cooking spray (check the ingredients), or line a baking sheet with foil.

3. Whisk up the two eggs in a large bowl.

4. In a separate bowl, mix the sugar, baking powder, and xanthan gum together.

5. Combine the peanut butter and the eggs and mix. Then add the sugar/baking powder/xanthan gum and mix until thoroughly combined.

6. Use a spoon or 1" ice cream scooper and drop dough onto cookie sheets about 2" to 3" apart.

7. Use a fork and press them down enough to make a textured surface.

8. Bake each batch for 15 minutes. Remove from oven, let cool for five minutes, then transfer the cookies to a wire rack.

Serves 12

Ingredients
2 large eggs
2 cups sugar
2 teaspoons baking powder (make sure it's gluten free; see recipe on page 93)
¼ teaspoon xanthan gum
2 cups peanut butter (natural/no sugar added is preferable)

Chapter 6
Finding a GI Doctor

"It's just gas." Maybe—but it could also be a sign of something more serious. When persistent gastrointestinal symptoms begin interfering with your daily life, such as interrupting work or sleep, you may need to seek the services of a medical professional trained to diagnose, treat, and prevent such problems. Gastroenterologists specialize in the prevention, diagnosis, and treatment of digestive tract and liver diseases. They also help you plan necessary exams and diagnostic tests to help you stay healthy.

When You Need Help

You might contact a gastroenterologist in cases of abdominal pain, rectal bleeding, or change in bowel habits when the diagnosis is unclear or where specialized diagnostic procedures are necessary. In fact, a gastroenterologist treats a broad range of conditions. Symptoms frequently evaluated by a gastroenterologist include:

- Chronic abdominal pain
- Persistent nausea and vomiting
- Persistent diarrhea
- Persistent constipation
- Unexplained rectal bleeding
- Persistent heartburn
- Painful or difficult swallowing
- Unexplained weight loss

Diseases typically treated by a gastroenterologist include gastroesophageal reflux disease (GERD), stomach or duodenal ulcers, Crohn's disease, pancreatitis, celiac sprue, intestinal polyps and cancers, irritable bowel syndrome, bile duct stones and tumors, and anemia from chronic intestinal bleeding.

Upper GI Symptoms

If your heartburn becomes more frequent than usual and is not relieved by over-the-counter medications, you need to see a physician. Potential problems include ulcers, gallbladder disease, or serious problems with your esophagus. Vomiting that goes on for more than twenty-four hours or is accompanied by persistent pain in the upper abdomen needs medical attention. It can signify anything from appendicitis or food poisoning to gallbladder disease or intestinal obstruction.

Lower GI Symptoms

Any major changes in your bowel habits warrant at least a call to your medical care provider. If you can't defecate, if you have persistent constipation, loss of bowel control, or bloody, tarry, or pale stools, then call your doctor. The possibilities range from food poisoning, irritable bowel syndrome, diverticulosis, or rarely, cancer.

Red Flags

Most of the time, you can call for an appointment and get it within a few weeks. If you are concerned about the wait, ask to be put on the cancellation list so they can call you at the last minute when someone cancels their appointment. However, if you experience GI symptoms accompanied by a sudden high fever, weight loss, blood in your stools, or vomiting, or pain severe enough that it consistently keeps you awake or prevents you from functioning, then you should simply go to your local emergency room.

Finding a Gastroenterologist

A gastroenterologist (GI) is a doctor who specializes in diagnosing and treating disorders of the entire gastrointestinal tract. Their field of study is called gastroenterology and includes all normal activity and disease of the digestive organs—everything from heartburn to colon cancer.

The American Board of Internal Medicine certifies most gastroenterologists and confirms they have received additional training in gastroenterology. Board-certified gastroenterologists must complete four years of college and four years of medical school and have received a medical degree to qualify. Then, the rigorous process includes another four to six years of specialty training in internal medicine and gastroenterology. After several years of clinical practice, the doctor must then complete an extensive series of examinations, or boards.

The Perfect Fit

Gastroenterologists sometimes specialize in certain parts of the digestive system, particular diseases, or patient groups. Subspecialties include:

- Pediatric gastroenterology
- Hepatology—Liver, gallbladder, pancreas, and the diseases that affect them

- Gastroenterology—Inflamatory bowel disease (IBD)
- Gastroenterology—Pancreaticobiliary jaundice
- Gastroenterology—Specialist upper GI

Once you've selected a physician, check out his credentials. You can contact the American Board of Medical Specialists at 1-866-ASK-ABMS (866-275-2267) or visit its website at *www.abms.org* to find out if your physician is board certified in at least one of the following areas:

- Internal medicine
- Gastroenterology
- Family practice
- Pediatrics (for patients who are children)

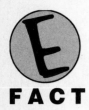

FACT

The American Gastroenterological Association has a website to help locate a GI doctor. You can search by last name, city, state, or zip code. The search results will list the names, addresses, and phone numbers for all physicians meeting your search criteria at *www.acg.gi.org/patients /phylocator.asp.*

If you are looking for a gastroenterologist, you may want to ask your family physician for a recommendation.

Referrals from Friends and Family

Word of mouth is a great way to find a good doctor. You want someone who has extensive experience with your type of concern. If someone you know has similar health issues, ask who their physician is and what their experience has been like.

Online Referrals

Random online searches for a health care provider may not net you the best results. However, a careful, intentional search may be helpful if you know what to look for. Just because a physician has a nifty website doesn't mean he or she is board certified in what you need.

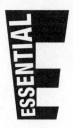

You may want to consider looking for a gastroenterologist affiliated with a teaching and research hospital. You may get a few more students tagging along for appointments and procedures, but if you have a particularly thorny case, access to the latest research and clinical trials might be helpful.

On the other hand, after spending a few hours online with a support group or other online forum where patients describe their experiences with their physicians, and the one you're considering keeps popping up as an excellent choice, then that's helpful to know.

Prepare for Your Appointment

Something isn't quite right. What used to work just fine, doesn't work. What didn't hurt, now does. Even if you are visiting the doctor for preventative care, you are responsible for making sure you get everything you need from your doctor and from this appointment.

Make the Call

Call the gastroenterologist's office to set up an appointment. If you are not a regular patient, don't even ask if they can go ahead and schedule a colonoscopy or other lab work. They won't. They need to meet you first, review your symptoms, and go from there. However, there may be some standard diagnostic testing, lab work, or stool samples, which typically occur at the first visit. Determine what you can't eat or drink prior to the appointment.

What to Bring with You

Ask your physician's office if there is anything in particular they will need you to bring. Your referring physician should forward the reason for the referral, as well as copies of recent laboratory results, X-ray reports, and so on, to the GI doctor. Allow plenty of time for the office to do so, but confirm a day or so before your appointment to make sure the information was received. Otherwise, plan on bringing along:

- A copy of your most recent insurance card
- Referral form (for your insurance needs)
- Recent lab work results and X-rays
- Food/symptom journal
- A list of medications you are currently taking and those you have taken in the past, along with notes about how well they worked and if side effects were a concern.

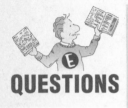

QUESTIONS

How do I get copies of my medical records from my primary care physician?
Records that come from other doctors' offices are the property of that physician's office, and only you can give authorization to have those records transferred. You must first sign a release form (available at your referring physicians' office or your specialist's) and ask that those records be sent to your new physician.

Decide on a Primary Objective

Prepare for your doctor's appointment in advance. Take the time to write down everything—your symptoms, allergies, medicines, previous medical procedures, conditions, and past diseases. Bring this information with you and show your gastroenterologist.

You may wish to ask a friend or family member to come to the appointment with you. Sometimes another set of ears can take notes or just make sure you don't miss valuable information.

Most people think they will remember everything the doctor says, but we often don't. Consider taking notes. Bring along a pen and paper and write down your gastroenterologist's answers.

During the visit, bring up your biggest concerns first. Let your gastroen-terologist know which symptoms bother you the most, and are affecting your lifestyle. Do not hesitate to talk about your feelings if your symptoms are causing you to feel worried, depressed, or embarrassed. Your emotions are a part of who you are.

The most important thing to bring with you is a brief, specific explanation of your current health concern. For example, "I know it's time for a checkup, and I wanted to know what tests I should have at my age." Do not say, "My stomach hurts." Instead, try "After I eat anything, I have severe cramping in my lower abdomen, and I feel nauseous for an hour afterward."

Insurance Coverage

Verify that your insurance covers the gastroenterologist or if they require a referral from your primary care physician. Use your insurance company's web-based search tool or call your insurance representative. Have the gastro-enterologist's office address and phone number ready.

Before you go in for your appointment, call your insurance company and find out what is covered and what you need to do for prior authorization. There may be some tests that will only be covered if ordered by a primary care physician, and not by a specialist, so find out first exactly what your plan covers.

Dealing with health insurance can be time-consuming, frustrating, and confusing, especially if you have a chronic health problem. You may be surprised to discover your plan will cover a variety of different treatment options, such as a pain management clinic or mental health professional, if your quality of life is severely impacted by your condition.

At Your Appointment

For your first appointment, expect to undergo a history and physical examination, review of records and X-rays, and discussion with the physician regarding diagnosis and treatment. To complete necessary paperwork, plan to arrive at least fifteen minutes early for your first visit. Many doctors have paperwork available online so you can fill it out and bring it with you.

Address Your Primary Concern First

This is the time to bring up the primary concern you have that you want addressed at this visit. Talk about your biggest concerns first. Let your gastroenterologist know about the symptoms that bother you the most, and do not hesitate to talk about your feelings.

Physical Exam

Expect to have your blood pressure taken and your height and weight measured. Most patients will be asked to partially disrobe and put on an examination gown.

The doctor will then interview you and perform a focused physical examination. Depending on the problem, this may include listening to the lungs and heart and examining the abdomen. Generally, the doctor will examine your abdomen by pressing in various places and feeling for any palpable abnormalities in your abdominal organs.

When medically appropriate, sometimes a simple digital rectal examination is performed. While a little uncomfortable, it only takes a few seconds and doesn't require any preparation. After the exam, your health care provider will discuss her assessment of your concerns and discuss what treatment or tests may be needed.

Take a Companion

If you are nervous, you may want to ask a family member to join you. Your companion can step out of the room during the physical exam and come back in when it is completed. When the doctor is explaining the diagnosis, what tests need to be done, and how to prepare for them, it can be helpful to bring along another set of ears.

Provide Specifics

Pain can be mild or pain can be excruciating. If you are not clear with your health care provider, he or she will not know how best to help you. If you hurt, describe where it hurts and how painful it is. Is the discomfort "aching," "throbbing," "sharp," or "burning"? Those specifics can help your gastroenterologist make assessments about the causes of your pain.

If you are taking medication, tell your gastroenterologist about any side effects you are experiencing. They may be typical or they may indicate that another medication might be a better treatment option. In the same way, as your symptoms change—either for better or worse—tell your gastroenterologist to help develop treatment that's best for you.

Be Honest

Do not be concerned with "keeping a stiff upper lip." This is not the time to suffer silently. Talk about the ways your discomfort is impacting your life. If you can't sleep because of heartburn, can't work because of diarrhea, or can't eat without doubling over in pain, it doesn't do you good if you don't share that information. No one is going to think you are any less of a person for not wanting to experience discomfort and pain. But you will risk getting an inaccurate diagnosis if you don't thoroughly and honestly explain your symptoms.

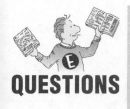

QUESTIONS

What is a physician's assistant, and why do I have to see him?
A physician's assistant (PA) is a health care provider licensed to practice medicine with the supervision of a physician. PAs practice as part of a team with the supervising physicians. They can perform physical exams, diagnose illnesses, carry out treatment plans, order and interpret lab tests, and provide patient education and preventive health care counseling. Think of him as another partner on your team!

Open Up

Talking about bowel habits may be embarrassing for you but certainly not for your gastroenterologist, who is relying on an accurate description to help with the diagnosis. When you see your health care provider, you will have a lengthy discussion about the status of your bowels. How often do you have a bowel movement? What do your feces normally look like? Is there mucus in your stool? When did the problem start? Where is the pain?

Your doctor has had many discussions with many patients about their bowel habits and problems and needs to know all of the information to make the most informed choice about diagnostic tests and treatment options. Don't let embarrassment keep you from getting the care you need and deserve. When it comes down to it, your digestive system is just another body part that everybody experiences difficulty with at some point.

Besides being open about your physical symptoms, you also need to be honest about lifestyle questions. Expect to be asked questions about your drinking, smoking, work, or family stress, and it is equally important to be honest with these questions. Again, you are not alone in your quest for better health, and you may be surprised to find your physician may have some helpful resources on your journey to better health.

Questions to Ask

Before you leave the office, make sure you know basic information. Ask these questions:

- What is the name of my condition? Are there any other names for it? (For example, gastroesophageal reflux disease [GERD] is also known as chronic heartburn.)
- How severe is my condition?
- Is my condition long-lasting (i.e., chronic)? Is it hereditary or related to my environment or lifestyle?
- What complications may I experience?
- Does my condition increase my risk for developing any other medical problems?

A Team Approach

Creating a partnership between you and your physician is important. Not only does it affect the quality of your care, but an uncomfortable relationship with your physician can also affect how well you will respond to treatment and how likely you will be to follow your doctor's advice.

You and your physician both have responsibilities in creating a good working relationship.

Your Role as Patient

You have an important role in being a part of a working team. To help in creating a good relationship with your physician, treat the doctor and office staff with courtesy and respect. When the doctor gives advice—even if it is unwanted lifestyle changes—follow it carefully. Ask for help if you need it, whether it's with quitting smoking, losing weight, or beginning an exercise program.

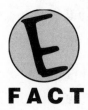

FACT

Studies confirm having a good doctor-patient relationship improves IBS. A study of 262 adult patients with IBS found 37 percent of those who received quality contact and discussion from their doctors reported moderate or substantial improvement in their disease, compared to other groups that received only observation.

Not every digestive problem has a quick fix, and your doctor may require time and tests to make a diagnosis. Part of your job is to give your health care provider enough time to accurately diagnose the problem.

Your Specialist's Role

You also have the right to have certain expectations of the members of your health care team. You need to be fully informed about your diagnosis and treatment options, including understanding the costs and risks of treatment. You have the right to have all of your questions answered and have a say in decisions affecting your health.

Your Family Doctor

Because the gastroenterologist provides specialized care in gastroenterology, you will still need your family doctor for other medical problems. In some cases, your primary care physician may monitor your digestive health issues, while others require long-term care with the GI doctor. Your specialist can send progress reports and test results to your primary care provider, but you will need to ask, sign release forms, and provide necessary contact information.

After the Visit

When you leave the doctor's office, you should have a good idea of what to do next. You may have instructions for diagnostic tests, a prescription for medication or lifestyle changes, or a referral to a professional better suited to help you.

Rarely, a physician will insist that symptoms are merely "in your head" and that you need to relax. While mental stress can impact your physical health, if you feel your concerns were dismissed too casually, then speak up.

Sometimes, a patient and a health care provider are simply not a good fit, even if the doctor was referred by someone you trust or is covered by your insurance company. For instance, if you are interested in complementary approaches, and the only tool in his arsenal is a prescription pad, you may want to consider finding a new provider. Or she may have a good reputation, but also has a horrible bedside manner. Decide what's important to you and ask yourself the following questions after your initial appointment:

- Was the physician respectful to me?
- Did the physician really listen to what I had to say?
- Did the physician spend a sufficient amount of time with me, or did I feel rushed during the appointment?
- Did the physician seem to have any useful suggestions?

If you feel good about the visit, you are on your way to developing a good patient/doctor relationship. If not, then you have the right to your medical records and test results, and you can change doctors or get a second opinion before you proceed.

Chapter 7
GI Tests

Often digestive disorders can be diagnosed with a physical exam and a careful history. Sometimes, diagnostic tests must be performed to rule out other diseases. While GI tests aren't enjoyable, they aren't usually painful, either. For many tests, some preparation will need to be done beforehand. Carefully preparing for a test makes it easier and more effective. Plus, once you know what to expect, you will feel more comfortable and know you are doing everything you can to maintain good digestive health.

When Tests Are Ordered

To protect your digestive health, you'll have to have some tests done. There's no way around it. Even if your physician is 99.9 percent sure of what's ailing you, you will still want to rule other problems out. Plus, some tests need to be done annually, whether because of your age, lifestyle, or other risk factors for certain diseases. Whether it's a quick physical exam or blood test, or more extensive diagnostic tests, here are the basics you need to know.

Test Preparation

Tests can be done in a hospital, special outpatient surgical center, or a physician's office. You will be asked to sign a form that verifies that you consent to having the procedure and that you understand what is involved.

Make sure you understand the answers to these questions:

- Will a board-certified gastroenterologist (specialist in diseases of the GI tract) be performing my diagnostic test?
- If not board certified, has my doctor completed a fellowship program or received special training in gastroenterology?
- About how many of these procedures has this doctor performed? About how many does the doctor perform each month?
- How should I prepare for this diagnostic test?
- How long will the test take?
- Will I be able to drive myself home immediately following the test?
- Are there any side effects or complications associated with this diagnostic test?
- If my test detects an abnormality, what will be the course of action? May abnormal tissue be removed during the procedure?
- How long will it take to get the results of the test? Should I call for the results, or will someone contact me?

Telephone number to call: _____

When to call: Date: _____ Time: _____

Blood Tests

The two most common blood tests are a *complete blood count* (CBC)—which measures the number of red blood cells, white blood cells, and platelets in the blood—and a basic metabolic panel (BMP). These screen for a variety of illnesses including: anemia, diabetes, kidney disease, liver disease, and an imbalance of certain minerals like sodium, potassium, and calcium (electrolytes). Two other frequently ordered tests will measure your cholesterol level and the function of your thyroid gland.

Blood tests can be performed on different parts of the blood, including:

- **Whole blood** (blood that has not been separated into its many components)
- **Blood plasma** (the liquid part of the blood)
- **Blood serum** (plasma that has had the clotting agent removed)
- **Blood cells** (the individual red blood cells, white blood cells, and platelets)

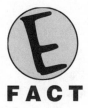

FACT

To get your blood flowing well, drink eight to ten glasses of liquid the day before and day of your test. It also makes the veins more likely to stick up and be found easily, so drink up for a day or two before your test. But remember to follow your doctor's instructions—some tests require that you not drink certain liquids prior to the test or that you avoid eating anything during the six hours before blood is drawn.

Differential

Also called white blood cell count (WBC), differential measures the number of white blood cells in a blood sample. This test also includes information about abnormal cell structure and the presence of immature cells.

Helicobacter Pylori Test

If you have symptoms of heartburn or a stomach ulcer, your doctor may order a blood test to determine if you have a stomach infection by a certain bacteria called *Helicobacter pylori*. The test checks to see if your immune system is creating antibodies to this bacterium. If the test is positive, you will need treatment to kill it.

Colonoscopies Are Critical

A colonoscopy is one of the best tools health care professionals have to detect colon cancer. It is an examination of your large intestine (colon) that allows the physician to view the entire length of the large intestine, and can often help identify abnormal growths, inflamed tissue, ulcers, and bleeding. It is most often used to look for early signs of cancer in the colon and rectum. It can also be used to look for causes of unexplained changes in bowel habits and to evaluate symptoms like abdominal pain, rectal bleeding, and weight loss.

Colonoscopy Preparation

The goal of colonoscopy prep is to eliminate all fecal matter from the colon so that the physician conducting the colonoscopy will have a clear view. Depending on your doctor, he will have very specific instructions about how to clean out your system.

You have thirty feet of digestive tract that needs to be thoroughly cleaned out. In order to remove all solid waste in the digestive tract quickly, it is necessary to cause diarrhea, leaving the colon clean. If waste is inside the colon when the procedure is performed, the physician may be unable to view the inside surface of the colon clearly. When the view of the colon surface is obscured, it can lead to a longer exam and can reduce its accuracy. It may also make it necessary for a second exam or could lead to remaining undiagnosed conditions.

Expect lots of loose stools, so plan to stay home the day and evening before your scheduled test. The cleanout process means that you will have many liquid bowel movements over several hours.

Colon Cleaning Products

An enema or oral laxatives will be prescribed to help you evacuate your bowels before a colon screening. The most common oral laxative (or lavage solution) requires you to drink four liters of nonabsorbable liquid. There are several different brands of the oral laxative solution. Which one you use depends on what your pharmacist has in stock, what your insurance company covers, and the flavor you prefer. They are all clear and come in a variety of flavors and unflavored. You can add some flavoring, like sugar-free lemonade mix, but don't add anything with bright colors or flavors, like cherry.

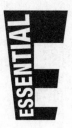

Be prepared. Buy the softest toilet paper you can find and use flushable wipes as needed. To avoid too tender of a bottom, you may want to apply petroleum jelly or 1 percent hydrocortisone cream after every bathroom stop.

You can also try a liquid diet to clean out your colon. The liquid diet should be clear and not contain food colorings, and may include:

- Fat-free bouillon or broth
- Strained fruit juice
- Water
- Plain coffee
- Plain tea
- Diet soda
- Gelatin

The Procedure

At the medical center, you'll change into a gown and you'll get an IV and an oxygen mask. You will probably have some form of sedative or anesthesia. You will be positioned on your left side during the procedure. The procedure itself only takes thirty to sixty minutes, but it is wise to plan on two to three hours for paperwork, waiting, preparation, and recovery.

During the procedure, the physician will insert a long, flexible, lighted tube called a colonoscope into your rectum. He will slowly guide it into the colon. The scope transmits an image of the inside of the colon which allows the physician to carefully examine its lining. In addition, the scope can blow air into the colon, inflating it to assist in visibility for the physician.

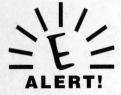

ALERT!

If you are taking blood-thinning medications, contact your prescribing physician for instructions. You may need to be off these drugs for one to ten days before the procedure, depending on the medicine.

The good thing about the procedure is that if anything abnormal is found, the physician can remove it at that time. Small instruments are passed through the scope and any removed tissue is sent to a lab for testing. If any bleeding occurs in the colon during the test, the doctor can pass a laser, heater probe, electrical probe, or special medicines through the scope to stop the bleeding. Very rarely, a polyp is too flat or big to remove during the procedure, and a separate surgery will need to be scheduled.

After the Procedure

You will be in the recovery room for about forty-five minutes to an hour after the procedure. A family member can usually be with you as you wait and can also hear the results of the test from the doctor. Afterward, you will probably have a dry mouth and feel drowsy and hungry. The dry mouth and drowsiness are from the sedation. It is an outpatient procedure, but you can't drive home afterward and you should take it easy the rest of the day.

Virtual Colonoscopies

Virtual colonoscopy (VC) uses a CT scanner to take a series of X-rays of the colon. Using a computer, it creates a three-dimensional view. A small tube is inserted in the rectum while a radiologist checks the images for suspicious polyps. The procedure is used to diagnose colon and bowel disease, including polyps, diverticulosis, and cancer. However, even with a VC, you still have to take the laxatives to clear out the bowels or it isn't a useful diagnostic tool. It is less expensive (about one-third the cost of a colonoscopy), but if you need to have a polyp removed, you'll have to have the colonoscopy done.

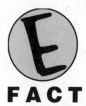

One study showed virtual colonoscopies were successful in detecting 90 percent of tumors at least 10 millimeters in diameter, although a standard colonoscopy would still be needed to remove the polyps.

Other Tests

In addition to a colonoscopy, there are other GI tests that may be ordered for you.

Rectal Exam

A rectal exam is the physical examination of the rectum, the last few inches of the bowel, just above the anus. You will need to remove or pull down your clothing from the waist down and lay on your side on an exam table with your knees pulled up toward your chest.

The first thing your doctor will do is conduct a visual examination of the anus and surrounding area to check for any rash, fissure, fistula, or as external or prolapsed hemorrhoids. An anoscope, a tube about three inches in length with light attached, might be used to do a visual examination of the rectum.

Sigmoidoscopy

A sigmoidoscope is a slender, hollow tube that is placed inside the colon. The scope has a tiny video camera that sends pictures to a TV screen and allows the physician to look at the inside of the large intestine from the rectum through the last part of the colon, called the sigmoid. It might be used to look for the cause of diarrhea, abdominal pain, or constipation, as well as early signs of cancer in the descending colon and rectum. It takes about fifteen minutes and doesn't usually require any medication.

Upper Endoscopy

An upper endoscopy uses a thin, flexible tube (endoscope) to look at the lining of the esophagus, stomach, and upper small intestine (duodenum). The procedure might be used to discover the reason for swallowing difficulties, nausea, vomiting, reflux, bleeding, indigestion, abdominal pain, or chest pain.

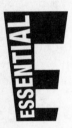

Before undergoing a test or procedure, you will be asked to give informed consent. The form is signed by the patient after the health care provider explains and describes the nature of the problem, alternative treatments, anticipated benefits of treatments, risks and side effects of treatments, and the consequences of no treatment.

During an intestinal endoscopy, the doctor inserts a tube into your small intestine and performs a biopsy. This procedure allows the physician to see abnormalities, like inflammation or bleeding, that do not generally show up well on X-rays. Just like during a colonoscopy, the physician passes instruments through the scope to treat bleeding abnormalities or remove samples of tissue (biopsy) for further tests.

When Body Imaging Tests Are Needed

Imaging tests, which include X-rays, sonograms (ultrasound), nuclear medicine scans, CT (computerized tomography), and MRI (magnetic resonance imaging), create pictures of internal body organs, tissues, structures, and pathways. Physicians will order such tests to help with the diagnosis of health conditions and the management of disease. They may also be used to assist during certain procedures and surgeries.

Starting with Abdominal Scans

Sonograms use high-frequency sound waves to create images of the shape and outline of various tissues and organs in the body. Abdominal X-rays provide basic information regarding the size, shape, and position of abdominal organs. Stones in the kidney, gallbladder, or ureters can also be seen with either sonograms or X-rays.

Upper or Lower GI Series or Barium Esophagram

An upper gastrointestinal (UGI) series looks at the upper and middle sections of the gastrointestinal tract (intestines). The test uses barium contrast material and X-ray fluoroscopy, which allows a "real-time" observation of what is occurring in this part of your digestive system. Before the test, you drink a mix of barium (barium contrast material) and water. Your doctor watches the movement of the barium through your esophagus, stomach, and the first part of the small intestine on a video screen. Several X-ray pictures are taken at different times and from different views.

MRI Tests

MRI stands for magnetic resonance imaging. The MRI is a noninvasive procedure that uses powerful magnets and radio waves to produce clear, cross-sectional or three-dimensional images of the body's tissues, even through bone and other obstructions. Lung, liver, pancreas, kidney, and spleen disorders may be seen with an MRI.

Nuclear Medicine Scans

Nuclear scans use radioactive substances and a special tool called a gamma camera to create images of organ systems in the body. A nuclear scan may be used to detect and diagnose digestive concerns such as diseases of the gallbladder, liver, or pancreas; gastrointestinal bleeding; or tumors.

CAT Scan

Computed axial tomography, also known as a CT scan, is a noninvasive and painless test that uses a rotating X-ray device to create detailed cross-sectional images of organs, bones, and other body parts. The illustrations produced by a CAT scan look as if you have been neatly sliced into sections and placed on display. CAT scans can detect appendicitis, inflammatory disorders of the bowel (including colitis), and abdominal tumors.

Taking Other Tests

Nobody enjoys providing a urine or stool sample, but a medical test conducted on a small sample collected from your body can give your doctor information that can help save or improve the quality of your life.

Fecal Occult Blood Test

A fecal occult blood test checks for hidden (occult) blood in the stool. It involves placing a very small amount of stool on a special card, which is then tested in the physician's office or sent to a laboratory. Your doctor may instruct you to avoid certain medications and follow certain dietary restrictions for several days before collecting the samples.

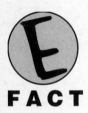

The American Cancer Society recommends that everyone age fifty and older get an annual fecal occult blood test and a colonoscopy at least every five to ten years.

Stool Culture

Providing a stool sample for labwork can be embarrassing. However, a stool culture can provide plenty of important information about your digestive health. The culture checks for the presence of abnormal bacteria in the digestive tract that may cause diarrhea and other problems. A small sample of stool is collected (usually by you at home in a specimen cup), then sent to a laboratory by your physician's office. It takes several days for the cultures to grow, but the tests will show whether abnormal bacteria are present. If there is bacteria in the stool, it will grow as colonies and look like dots on the surface of the gel. Each bacteria has its own unique fingerprint, so to speak, and laboratory technicians will look at the physical characteristics of the colonies—their shape, color, and some of their chemical properties—to determine which bacteria have taken up home in your colon.

Chapter 8
Lubricate Your Body

Clean water is one of the most important needs of your body. The amount of water in your body will impact your long-term health. On a normal day, you can lose up to a half gallon of water per day just in normal perspiration, urination, and breathing. How your body functions is, in part, dependent on how efficiently fluids are utilized and distributed. Make sure you're filling up your body with what it needs and craves!

Water and Your Body

After oxygen, water is the human body's most important need. Water carries waste products and toxins from the body, actively participates in many chemical reactions, acts as a lubricant and cushion around joints, serves as a shock absorber inside the eyes and spinal cord, aids in the body's temperature regulation, and helps maintain blood volume.

Water Protects Your Overall Health

If you do not get enough fluid, you will not feel well. After all, you can live without food for a month, but only a week without water. A common cause of daytime fatigue is inadequate fluid intake. Researchers suspect that 75 percent of Americans have mild, chronic dehydration.

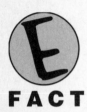

FACT

You need water because so much of your makeup is water! The average adult contains 40 to 50 quarts or 10 to 13 gallons of water. Blood is 83 percent water, muscles 75 percent, brain 75 percent, heart 75 percent, bones 22 percent, lungs 86 percent, kidneys 83 percent, and eyes 95 percent.

Clinical studies show that drinking eight glasses of water a day can decrease the risk of colon cancer and bladder cancer, and may reduce the risk of breast cancer. Preliminary research suggests drinking eight to ten glasses of water a day can ease back and joint pain for up to 80 percent of sufferers.

Water Aids in Digestion

Healthy digestion requires adequate fluid intake. The colon is your body's fluid regulator. If you're not drinking enough, your colon steals water from the waste material and gives it to the body, causing the stools to be water deprived or hard. These hard, dry stools are difficult to pass, because they stick to the dry wall of the colon.

By drinking plenty of water each day, you help your body stay hydrated enough, so that it doesn't need to extract much water at all from the solid waste materials that are moving through the colon. Since the waste material keeps its water, it stays soft and pliable so that it's able to move through the colon at a much easier and faster rate.

One of the important jobs of water is to help your kidneys remove wastes like uric acid, urea, and lactic acid. If you do not have enough water to dissolve the wastes then they cannot be removed effectively and you run the risk of kidney damage.

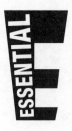

We dehydrate as we get older. Because the thirst response declines with aging, seniors don't get as thirsty as younger people and must make an effort to drink water even when not thirsty. To try to fill the basic requirements of one-half to two-thirds of your body weight in ounces of water per day, seniors should remember to sip throughout the day.

Water Intake Guidelines

The gold standard has always been that everybody needs eight glasses a day. That isn't the best guide. Most people should increase their water consumption, but individual needs vary. Your personal water needs are influenced by your physical activity level; consumption of meat, eggs, or salty foods; fever; heat; or dry, hot, or windy climates.

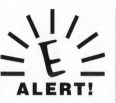

One way of getting enough fluid is to up your vegetable and fruit intake. Many vegetables are more than 90 percent water, and many other foods, like legumes and grains, are more than 80 percent water after being cooked. Of course, soups and broths are nearly all water.

A basic guideline for how much water you need is to divide your weight in half and then consume that many ounces of water each day. So a 128-pound person needs 64 ounces, but a 160-pound person needs 80 ounces. These guidelines are for total fluid intake, including fluid from all food and beverages. How does your total fluid intake compare?

Prevent Dehydration

By sweating, urinating, and breathing, your body gets rid of about ten cups of fluid a day. When you get rid of fluid, you also dump electrolytes, which are minerals like sodium and calcium that keep your body's fluids balanced. If you exercise, mow the lawn, or forget to drink as much water as you should (e.g., during a long airplane flight), your body will become dehydrated.

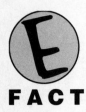

Poor hydration can harm a child's mental performance and learning ability. Symptoms of mild dehydration may include tiredness, headaches, and a feeling not unlike jet lag, as well as reduced alertness and ability to concentrate. Encourage your child's school to allow plenty of water breaks, or ideally a personal water bottle at every desk.

Even becoming mildly dehydrated (when you lose as little as 1 percent to 2 percent of your body weight) can seriously impact your body's ability to function. It is fairly easy to become dehydrated. In fact, by the time you become thirsty, your body is telling you it's dehydrated!

Mild dehydration signs include:

- Thirst
- Flushed face
- Dry, warm skin
- Lightheadedness or dizziness made worse when you stand
- Weakness
- Cramping in the arms and legs
- Having few or no tears
- Headache
- A lack of energy
- Dry mouth and tongue with thick saliva

Choose Your Water Carefully

There is no perfect water filter or purifying system to eliminate every single potentially harmful element in our water. Compared to much of the world, however, water in North America meets most safety guidelines. The United States Environmental Protection Agency (EPA) sets guidelines to measure water standards, with the goal of making sure our water is safe. Take responsibility for learning about where your water comes from, how it is filtered, and what you can do to ensure its safety.

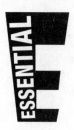

What color is your urine? Instead of relying on thirst as an indicator, check the color of your urine. If you're well hydrated, your urine will be clear or light colored. If not, your urine will be dark yellow or amber.

City Water Toxins

Tap water, in particular, always contains more than just water. Tap water is known to often be contaminated with toxic heavy metals like lead or cadmium or with fluoride, which is associated with an increased risk of cancer, digestive disorders, and kidney disease. One reason is that a number of different chemicals are added to city water to both stabilize the water and to keep the pipes from rusting.

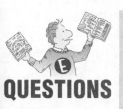

I have questions about my drinking water; whom should I call?
A good place to start is the Environmental Protection Agency's Safe Drinking Water Hotline: 1-800-426-4791. It's free and offers information on local drinking water quality, drinking water standards, public drinking water systems, and wells.

An area's water table can become contaminated in a number of different ways. Industrial chemicals and wastes, pesticides, and other farm chemicals often seep through the soil to contaminate the water table. Even though the individual chemicals are bad enough, volatile chemicals (those hydrocarbons that readily vaporize) can combine with other chemicals (like chlorine) and form even more toxic products.

Well Water Risks

Getting your water from a well has its own concerns. According to the CDC, contaminated private well water causes one-fourth of the drinking water outbreaks that make people sick. Runoff pollutants can also seep into groundwater, and microorganisms, heavy metals, lead, copper, household waste, fluoride, and more can all be found in traces in ground water. If it's in the groundwater, it's in your well.

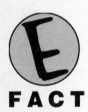

FACT

You should have your well water tested regularly, but do it sooner if there are known problems with well water in your area, you have experienced problems near your well (i.e., flooding, land disturbances, and nearby waste disposal sites), or you replace or repair any part of your well system.

If you are a homeowner with a private well, you should test your well water annually to make sure you've got safe drinking water. Contact your health or environmental department, or a private laboratory to test for germs and harmful chemicals. The CDC recommends testing for fecal coliform, nitrates, volatile organic compounds, and pH levels. If you live near farm animals, heavy industrial sites, or commercial agriculture fields, you may be at a higher risk for pollutants.

Water Bottle Risks

Bottled water's popularity is fueled in part by suspicions over the quality of tap water. You may not be getting what you pay for. Even though the label may say pure, bottlers are required in most cases only to meet the same quality standards as tap water. In one survey of 103 brands of bottled water, one-third of the brands contained unsafe levels of contamination, including synthetic organic chemicals, bacteria, and arsenic.

The report showed that the contents of one bottle came from an industrial parking lot next to a hazardous waste site. Ironically, the bottle was labeled "spring water." However, the FDA does now insist that bottled water must come from a spring if the bottler claims that it does.

Even if you are drinking spring water, the bottle might make you sick. The other concern about bottled water is the plastic used to make the bottles. Most plastic bottles contain bisphenol A (BPA). In laboratory animals, low-dose exposure to BPA has been linked to cancer, diabetes, fertility problems, and behavior disorders. If you need to use plastic, look for No. 1 PETE, No. 2 HDPE, No. 4 LDPE, or No. 5 PP, and refuse the rest.

Water Filters

Regardless of whether your water comes from a well or the city, add a water filter system. Most personal water filters are charcoal activated. That means that when charcoal is initially processed, it becomes very absorptive. When used in a water filter, it absorbs sediments and particulates that we want eliminated from our water. Popular pour-through water filters use charcoal to remove sediment. Charcoal water filters are inexpensive, effective, and do not waste much water.

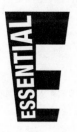

Warm water with lemon is a soothing digestive tonic. Heat 8 to 10 ounces water, add the juice of a lemon, and honey to taste. For a little variation, use lime instead of lemon juice, or add a slice of fresh ginger or a mint or basil leaf.

Beverages to Limit

Just because it's liquid, doesn't mean it's helpful. Every time you choose a glass of soda or a cup of coffee, for example, you are robbing your body of valuable nutrients. For example, caffeine leaches calcium from your bones.

Plus, depending on the drink, you might be adding more risks to your digestive health.

Kick the Caffeine

Coffee has well-documented side effects: anxiety, insomnia, tremors, and irregular heartbeat. It can also irritate the digestive system, bladder, and prostate. Coffee consumption of more than one cup per day appears to increase the risk of hypertension. Even decaffeinated coffee has some caffeine in it. Keep your intake to no more than 300 mg of caffeine per day.

Avoid Alcohol

For most people, an occasional drink of alcohol is not harmful. However, there are few benefits, and some people with digestive health issues should avoid it entirely. Many people with GERD and IBS find that drinking even small amounts of alcohol can be irritating. Alcohol can affect the lining of the gastrointestinal tract and cause nausea, vomiting, and diarrhea.

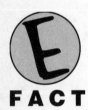

National health guidelines call for men to have no more than two alcoholic drinks a day and women to have no more than one. One alcoholic drink is the equivalent of 4 ounces of wine, 10 ounces of a wine cooler, 12 ounces of beer, or 1¼ ounces of distilled liquor, such as whiskey, vodka, or scotch.

If you choose to drink, avoid mixed drinks with sour mixes or strong juices like tomato, orange, or grapefruit juices. They can lead to reflux. Although the potential benefits of red wine for the heart have been widely touted, most people are not aware that some grapes provide the same apparent benefits. Plus, you don't have to take the risks involved with consuming the alcohol. In addition, grapes are better for you. They contain the beneficial polyphenols found in wine that are linked to a preventive role for the main chronic diseases such as cancer and cardiovascular and all inflammatory disease.

Fruit Juice

Juices provide nutrients in a form from which they are readily absorbed by the body. They are also a healthy way to get the water your body needs. Fruit juices have benefits, like vitamin C in orange juice and fiber in prune juice. However, fruit juices also tend to be high in sugar. If you can adapt to the somewhat stronger flavors, vegetable juices are better for you and much lower in sugar. If you drink juice, buy organic, because the same pesticides found in grapes and apples don't go anywhere when made into fruit juice.

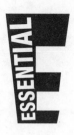

Ayurveda recommends avoiding cold drinks at meals and ice cold foods in general. Iced water, normally served at restaurants, extinguishes the digestive fire. Even juice or milk right out of the refrigerator is too cold for the digestion. Juice should be taken at room temperature and water without ice.

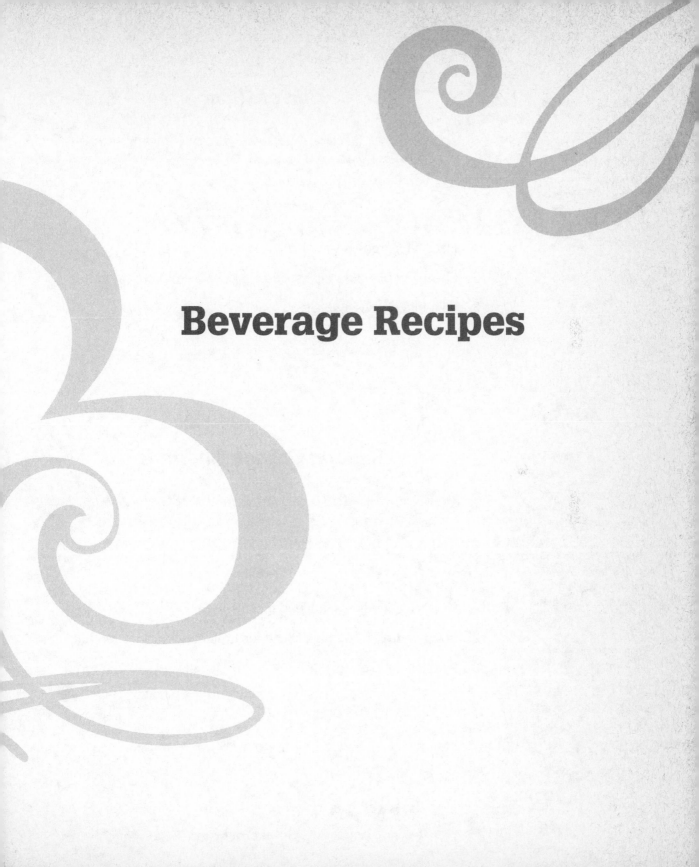

Beverage Recipes

Carrot Shake

Serves 2

Ingredients
1 cup carrot juice
1 cup fat-free yogurt
2 teaspoons vanilla extract
½ ripe banana, sliced
¼ teaspoon nutmeg
2 ice cubes

Carrot juice is a great source of vitamin A and B complex vitamins. Its mineral content is equally rich and includes calcium, copper, magnesium, potassium, sodium, phosphorus, chlorine, sulfur, and iron.

1. Place all ingredients in blender container.

2. Cover and blend on high speed for 1 minute, or until smooth.

3. Pour into glasses and serve.

Banana Orange Smoothie

Serves 2

Ingredients
1½ cups yogurt, plain or
    vanilla, low fat
½ cup orange juice
¼ cup wheat germ
½ teaspoon vanilla
1 large banana, sliced
1 tablespoon honey or rice
    syrup
½ teaspoon cinnamon or
    nutmeg

Wheat germ is a good source of vitamin B and also helps in digestion, healthy skin, and repair of tissues. Wheat germ is also a great source of natural fiber, which helps prevent constipation.

1. Place all ingredients in blender container.

2. Cover and blend on high speed for 1 minute, or until smooth.

3. Pour into glasses and serve.

Fruity Protein Drink

Soy helps to dissolve gallstones after they have formed, and may even prevent their formation. It may even assist in the prevention of kidney disease.

1. Place all ingredients in blender container.

2. Cover and blend on high speed for 1 minute, or until smooth.

3. Pour into a glass and serve.

Serves 1

Ingredients
3 tablespoons soy protein
    (powder)
¼ banana
¼ cup apple juice
3–4 ounces soy or rice milk

Tropical Smoothie

Mangos are great to combat acidity and poor digestion and are often recommended for constipation. Mangos contain phenols, the phenolic compound thought to have powerful antioxidant and anticancer abilities.

1. Arrange banana, mango, and pineapple in single layer on baking sheet.

2. Cover and freeze until fruit is frozen solid, about 2 hours.

3. Place all ingredients in blender container.

4. Cover and blend on high speed for 1 minute, or until smooth.

5. Pour into glasses and serve immediately.

Serves 2

Ingredients
1 very ripe banana, sliced
1 cup diced, pitted, peeled
    fresh mango (from about
    1 small mango)
1 cup diced, peeled fresh
    pineapple
1 cup unsweetened pineapple
    juice
½ cup canned light
    unsweetened coconut
    milk
1 teaspoon fresh lime juice

Iced Nettle Tea

Serves 4

Ingredients
1 quart water
2 tablespoons dry nettle leaves
Lemon juice or sweetener to taste

Nettle is detoxifying and improves the ability of the liver and kidneys to cleanse the blood. It also curbs the appetite and cleanses toxins from the body. It is also used as an analgesic, anti-inflammatory, antiseptic, blood cleaner, diuretic, and digestive stimulant. Nettle leaves can be ordered online or in many specialty health food stores.

1. Bring a quart of water to a boil.

2. Put 2 tablespoons of dry nettle leaves into a teapot and cover with the boiling water.

3. Let the tea brew for 3 to 5 minutes.

4. Strain before cooling.

5. Add more water, lemon, and your favorite sweetener.

Indian Lassi

Serves 2

Ingredients
2 cups plain yogurt
1 cup hot and 2 cups cold water
2 tablespoons raw cane sugar
2 drops rosewater (optional)
Pinch of ground cardamom
Fruit that can be well blended, like berries or bananas

With protein, calcium, magnesium, riboflavin, vitamins B-6 and B-12, and more, plain low-fat or nonfat yogurt is better for you than skim milk because of the good bacteria in it. A lassi is a yogurt shake, often served after a meal to aid in digestion.

Blend all ingredients together on low speed just enough to mix, or use a blender stick or whisk.

Hot Pomegranate Cider

The sweet, tart, and juicy taste of the pomegranate is a staple in Mediterranean and Middle Eastern cooking. It's hard to eat raw, but its juice has antioxidant properties three times greater than those of green tea.

1. Pour pomegranate and apple juices into a slow cooker and turn the heat to low.

2. Place cinnamon stick, cloves, orange zest and cranberries in cheesecloth bag and add to juice.

3. Add vanilla and honey, then simmer for 1 hour, stirring occasionally.

4. When cider begins to steam, it's ready to serve. Taste it at this point to make sure it's sweet enough and remove bag.

Serves 8–10

Ingredients
1 quart pomegranate juice
2 quarts apple juice
1 cinnamon stick
6–8 whole cloves
½ cup dried cranberries
½ teaspoon pure vanilla extract
⅔ cup honey
1 teaspoon orange zest

Blueberry Splash

To juice the pomegranate, cut it in half (as you would a grapefruit) and juice using a citrus reamer or a juicer. Pour mixture through a cheesecloth-lined strainer or sieve. One large pomegranate will produce about ½ cup of juice.

1. Place all ingredients in blender container.

2. Cover and blend on high speed for 1 minute, or until smooth.

3. Pour into glasses and serve.

Serves 2

Ingredients
½ cup pomegranate juice
6 ounces fat-free blueberry yogurt, frozen
1 cup fresh blueberries
1 cup nonfat milk
1 teaspoon vanilla extract
Honey, to taste
Handful of crushed ice

Sweet Beet Juice

Serves 2

Ingredients
5 carrots, peeled and
    chopped
1 apple peeled, cored, and
    diced
½ beet, peeled and chopped

Purchase firm, rock-hard beets. As a root, they can be stored for months in the refrigerator. Beets are also high in minerals that strengthen the liver and gallbladder and form the building blocks for blood corpuscles and cells.

1. Place all ingredients in food processor.

2. Cover and blend on high speed for 1 minute, or until smooth.

3. Pour into glasses and serve.

Tart Cherry Smoothie

Serves 1

Ingredients
½ cup frozen tart cherries
¼ cup cherry juice
¼ peeled banana
¼ cup crushed pineapple

Fruits such as pineapple and papaya are full of enzymes to aid digestion, while the anthocyanins in black cherries have been proved to reduce the risk of colon cancer significantly.

1. Place all ingredients in blender.

2. Cover and blend on high speed for 1 minute, or until smooth.

3. Pour into a glass and serve.

Chapter 9
Bacteria Balancing Act

Your body is host to about 100 trillion microbes, most in your colon, where they live and grow, aid in digestion, and prime the immune system. More than 400 different types of bacteria live in the gastrointestinal tract alone. Most of these bacteria are not harmful, and some are actually beneficial and important for normal growth and development. Under normal circumstances, the "good" bacteria far outnumber the bad, but any shift in the balance of bacteria may affect how well your gastrointestinal tract functions.

The Microbe Dance

The small intestine is approximately twenty feet long and is lined with millions of tiny villi, which are like fingers or projections with the primary responsibility for the absorption of nutrients. If you were to flatten out the villi and the small intestinal wall, it would stretch as wide as a tennis court. This enormous surface area is devoted to assimilation. Digested food, or "chyme," and fiber make up about 60 percent of the mass that travels through the intestinal tract. The rest of the volume is made up of mucus and bacteria. Which kind of bacteria there is has everything to do with your health.

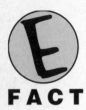

FACT

Metabolomics—the study of metabolites and other chemicals produced by the body and its bacteria—is one of the fastest-growing biomedical niches. Researchers suggest bacteria could play a role in neurological disorders such as attention-deficit hyperactivity disorder, Tourette's syndrome, and autism.

Bad Bacteria

While most people have heard of peptic ulcers, they may not have heard of the organism behind it. The disease-causing bacterium *Helicobacter pylori* is actually the culprit. Ulcers aren't the only problem with bacteria. Researchers are beginning to link obesity and nonalcoholic liver disease with other types of intestinal bacteria.

If you don't have enough friendly bacteria, it means your intestinal microflora is out of balance. So what? Without enough friendly bacteria, your overall health is affected. How else can you combat the bad, or pathogenic, bacteria like salmonella, klebsiella, clostridia, giardia (waterborne parasite), shigella (dysentery), or staphylococcus (infection)? Whenever healthy bacteria are diminished, bodies become threatened by opportunistic bacteria, other parasites, fungi, and candida (yeast). Modern food processing leaves very few of the good-guy bacteria behind.

Good Bacteria

Probiotics decrease inflammation in the gut, can help provide nutrition needed for healthy gut lining cells to synthesize vitamins such as the B vitamins biotin and folate, and can break down certain cancer-causing chemicals (carcinogens) in our diet. Probiotics decrease responses to both food allergens and pollen allergens.

Another advantage of probiotics is that they are believed to produce anti-bacterial substances, which render harmless or kill hostile bacteria. The probiotics are able to do so by changing the area's levels of acidity. In doing so, it deprives the disease-causing bacteria of their nutrients.

Probiotics produce natural antibiotics (acidophilus produces the antibiotic acidophilin) and can reduce or prevent infections in the gut. Probiotics are commonly prescribed now to prevent or treat *Clostridium difficile* bacterial infection, a common complication of antibiotic therapy.

Produce More Vitamins

Good bacteria manufacture some of the B vitamins, including niacin (B_3), pyridoxine (B6), folic acid, and biotin. Plus, they manufacture the milk-digesting enzyme lactase which helps digest dairy products.

Protect Against Cancer

Many researchers believe that interactions between diet, the intestinal microflora, and the cells in the lining of the colon, together with genetic factors, may be what causes colon cancer to develop. Healthy bacteria may help maintain a healthy intestinal microflora and promote a healthy environment. Another theory for the cause of colon cancer is that prolonged exposure to cancer-causing compounds in the colon may trigger the process.

Protect Your Intestines

When intestinal function is altered, it may increase the risk for developing certain chronic intestinal disorders such as colon cancer, Crohn's disease, ulcerative colitis, irritable bowel syndrome, and diarrhea. Probiotics have been shown to have a detoxifying effect in the colon. Prevention of diarrhea is the most frequently touted health claim for probiotics.

Creating Imbalance

All of us have more than a trillion microbes and more than 1,000 different types of bacteria in our body. Each of our collections of microbes or flora is as unique as our fingerprint. Our unique gut flora "fingerprint" is extremely stable over our lifetime, becoming established early in childhood and generally remaining unchanged until old age unless disrupted by antibiotics. Over time, the types and number of bacteria are influenced by several factors, including stress, antibiotics, illness, aging, and your diet.

Dietary Reactions

Your intestinal bacterial health is immediately affected by the type of diet you eat. Your healthy intestinal bacteria thrive on a diet that focuses on complex carbohydrates like vegetables, whole grains, and beans and limits animal fats, fatty meat, and sugars. The good news is that a diet that is healthy for overall health is also best for healthy bacteria.

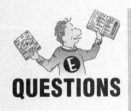

QUESTIONS

Will eating probiotics interfere with the efficacy of antibiotics?
Some physicians recommend acidophilus (for the small intestine) and bifidobacteria (for the large intestine) concurrently whenever antibiotics are prescribed. Antibiotics are assimilated so quickly into your body that probiotics will not interefere with how well they work.

Problems with Antibiotics

Keeping a stable healthy gut flora is becoming more difficult because of overuse of antibiotics, especially those given inappropriately for viral infections or those found in food. In addition, more powerful antibiotics are being given for infections due to increasingly resistant bacteria.

While antibiotics are great for getting rid of the bad bacteria, they kill off the good bacteria, too. During the course of antibiotics, research shows that certain probiotics can reduce antibiotic-induced diarrhea by 20 percent. Especially after a round of antibiotics, commit to two servings of probiotic-friendly food a day for at least a week.

Effects of Stress

The amount of stress in your life and how you handle it may also have an effect on the bacteria balance in your GI tract. Long-term (or chronic) stress is worse for your health than short-term (or acute) stress. Irritable bowel syndrome and inflammatory bowel disease (such as Crohn's disease and ulcerative colitis) are very closely related to stress. Another concern with long-term stress is that it also has the ability to sensitize the gut, which may then produce allergies to specific foods.

Fix the Imbalance

Every day there is new evidence emerging of the health benefits of probiotics and/or new diseases being linked to altered gut flora (dysbiosis). Just a few of the diseases or conditions linked to altered gut flora which may be improved by taking probiotics include dental cavities, Crohn's disease, ulcerative colitis, celiac disease, diabetes, heart disease, allergies, intestinal infections, yeast infections (especially vaginal), colds and respiratory infections, rheumatologic conditions, multiple sclerosis, autism, and cancer.

Adding Bacteria

One common analogy used to discuss healthy bacteria balance is the idea of a garden that has been overgrown with weeds, or bad bacteria. As any gardener knows, you can't just add new plants to a weedy garden. First, weeds must be pulled and the good seeds planted. In time, good plants will take over. In the same way, lactic acid bacteria, such as acidophilus and bifidobacterium, are the good weeds which have to overtake the other bacteria. But the bad weeds of parasites and candida must be reduced so that the gut wall can heal.

Decoding the Bacteria

The term *friendly bacteria* is used to describe the types of bacteria that offer some benefit when ingested. Bacteria make the holes in swiss cheese and give buttermilk a tangy flavor. But how are you supposed to know what to take? With thousands of different types, it can be hard to know the difference.

What are the differences between strains? *L. casei*, a common probiotic, has been commonly studied, and certain strains, like *L. casei* DN-114001 and *L. casei* Shirota, have been found beneficial. Some corporations, like Dannon, have even trademarked their own unique strains, like *L. casei* Immunitas. According to company spokespeople, the differences between strains can be compared to the differences between Chihuahuas and German shepherds. They might both be dogs, but their abilities are significantly different.

Adding Probiotics

Probiotics are live microorganisms that have been shown to have a beneficial health effect on the body. They must contain a sufficient number of these friendly bacteria that are still alive and active at the end of the shelf-life of the product and be proven to survive the strong acids in the stomach. There are no known side effects of probiotics. When consumed, they gradually become part of the healthy bacteria that normally live in the digestive system.

Understanding Prebiotics

Prebiotics are substances ingested to promote the growth of probiotics. Two of the most commonly used prebiotics are inulin and fructo-oligosaccharides (FOS). Synbiotics are supplements or functional foods that contain both a prebiotic and a probiotic.

Probiotics Basics

Not all live microorganisms or live culture bacteria like those in fermented foods or yogurt have been shown to have a health benefit to qualify as probiotics. You can add a wide variety of different types of probiotics to your diet through food, beverages, and even supplements.

Probiotics in Beverages

What if you can't stand yogurt? For some people, the texture just doesn't feel right. If that's your problem, then consider a drinkable yogurt. Several companies make them in a variety of flavors. Usually packaged in three- to six-ounce bottles, the taste is similar to a thin milk shake. Look for all-natural, fruit-flavored smoothie drinks to get two servings of fruit and a day's recommended daily allowance of vitamin C.

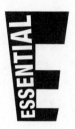

For something completely different, consider kombucha, a fermented tea drink. Usually, tea, water, and sugar are combined together and heated gently, then starter cultures are introduced into the mixture, exactly as is done with yogurt or kefir.

Another product similar to drinkable yogurt is kefir, a probiotic-laden drink made with animal or plant milk. Kefir comes in a wide range of flavors, but usually contains lactose. There are kefir drinks for kids, but watch out for sugar content and artificial colors. The advantage? It offers a wider variety of different strains of probiotics. It is also made into cheeses. If you are looking for another probiotic drink, consider lassi. Lassi is a popular Indian drink, perhaps best described as a cultured-milk smoothie (see recipe on page 132).

Probiotics in Food

Keep your eyes on grocery shelves as food manufacturers seek ways to include probiotic bacteria in products like nutrition bars, juice, and cereal. The good news? Probiotic-infused chocolate bars and frozen yogurt have already hit the market!

Here's one warning: Probiotics are good for the body, but there's a lot we still don't know. We don't know how much we need or even which strands. Incorporating probiotics in a healthy diet is a smart thing to do, but don't throw good nutrition out the window to do it. If you're going to treat yourself with a specialty probiotic food, make sure you don't add other things into your diet that you don't want—like high-fructose corn syrup.

When deciding how much of what kind to incorporate, Dr. Miguel Freitas, PhD, director of scientific affairs for Dannon Company, makes these suggestions:

First, look for a company you know and trust. Then go back to clinical evidence. If the particular strain on the package has scientific proof that it works, then you should be able to find it. Look on the package, and you should be directed to the company's website. The website should be clear and provide access to clinical studies in a way you would understand.

Shopping for Probiotics

How many billions of bacteria do you need? Scientists aren't sure of exact numbers. But it isn't even easy to know what number to look for. Due to the vast number of cells involved in probiotics, counts for these bacteria in any product tend to be very high, often numbering in the billions. The numbers are sometimes expressed as a CFU (or colony forming unit) count. But what your yogurt has today may be different tomorrow. As dairy products age, the culture count lessens, sometimes significantly.

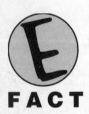

If you are trying to limit food in plastic containers because you are concerned about chemicals in plastics leaching into your food, a few yogurt companies share your concern. Some now sell yogurt in larger, glass containers. You may have to order them online and have it shipped, but for peace of mind, it may be worth it.

Not all yogurts contain probiotics. While all yogurts require live bacteria in their starter cultures, they don't have to be viable in the finished product. *L. acidophilus* is the most commonly added bacteria. The National Yogurt Association (NYA) has developed a "Live & Active Cultures" seal that requires refrigerated yogurt to contain at least 100 million cultures per gram at the time of manufacture, and frozen yogurt to contain at least 10 million cultures per gram at the time of manufacture. Don't use it as a shopping guide, because it measures the amount the product started with, not how much was left at the end. While you're looking at the label, avoid yogurt that says "heat treated after culturing" on the label. This means that it was pasteurized, a process that destroys live cultures.

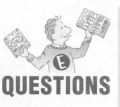

QUESTIONS

What if my kids don't like yogurt?
Pour drinkable yogurt into ice cube trays or small paper drinking cups. If you are using regular yogurt, combine two cups with enough milk to smooth it out and shake a few times, then pour. Add a popsicle stick, freeze and you have a yummy popsicle or fun cubes to use in milk. Enjoy!

Bacteria in Supplements

What's wrong with choosing a probiotic supplement? You are getting the good bacteria, but you are also missing out on some other important nutrients you might get otherwise. For example, fermented dairy products like yogurt are great source of calcium, riboflavin, vitamin B12, and potassium. They also provide amino acids, which have been found to be important nutrients for good health. Plus, even the fermenting process creates healthy byproducts, including functional peptides (amino acids smaller than a protein), which researchers believe may have beneficial effects.

Chapter 10
Food Safety

Nearly 100 million cases of food-related illness and several thousand food-related deaths happen each year in the United States. The dangers of food-borne disease are on the rise. In fact, you might even have been a victim of food-related illness and not even known it. From the time a product is made to the time it enters your mouth, there are dozens of opportunities for contamination. Here's what you can do to protect yourself and your family.

Recognize Food-Borne Disease

Food-borne diseases are the greatest food-related danger you face after poor eating habits. Toxins and infectious agents find their way into our food supply when produce is sprayed with bad water; when sick animals are butchered; or when stores, restaurants, or individuals prepare or store food badly. With more than 600 food-borne diseases, virtually everything you eat—from fast-food hamburgers to grocery store strawberries—can harbor disease-causing organisms. Throughout the course of human history, tiny food-borne microorganisms have killed more people than all wars and natural disasters combined.

Symptoms of Food Poisoning

When you ingest contaminated food, the microorganisms irritate and inflame the gastrointestinal tract. The most common symptoms of food-borne illness include abdominal pain, diarrhea, and vomiting. In extremely severe cases, illness can progress and lead to high fevers, internal hemorrhaging, kidney failure, and even death.

Illness Time Frame

Food-borne illness can affect one person, or it can occur as an outbreak in a group of people who all ate the same contaminated food. Symptoms of food poisoning can begin in as little as half an hour after ingesting contaminated food. What can make it difficult to identify a food-borne illness is that some toxins do not cause symptoms for up to thirty-six hours after ingestion. By then, you may have forgotten what you ate and assume you are coming down with the flu.

Secondary Illnesses

What many people do not realize is that some cases of food-borne illnesses leave something behind. Known as sequela, it is a disease or condition that results from an original disease. Another way of referring to it is a long-term complication. Scientists are just now beginning to understand long-term chronic illness as a characteristic of some food-borne diseases. Food-borne bacteria have been proven to cause arthritic disorders, such as Guillian-Barre Syndrome, meningitis, and hemolytic uremic syndrome, which is often fatal in infants and young children.

Who's at Risk?

No one is immune to food-borne illness. For example, even if you are in excellent health, undercooked eggs have the potential to make you sick. But some people are at higher risk for food-borne illness, especially older adults, pregnant women, very young children, and people with weakened immune systems. As such, high risk groups must take extra precautions with their diet. An immune system may be compromised by medical treatments like chemotherapy or by chronic illnesses like AIDS, cancer, diabetes, or liver or kidney disease.

High-risk individuals should not eat:

- Soft-cooked or runny eggs
- Caesar salad dressing
- Hollandaise sauce
- Raw or rare hamburger
- Carpaccio (thin shavings of raw beef fillet)
- Beef or steak tartare
- Raw fish: sushi, sashimi, ceviche, tuna carpaccio
- Raw molluscan shellfish: raw clams, oysters, mussels, scallops
- Refrigerated pâté or meat spreads
- Refrigerated smoked seafood
- Deli salads
- Unpasteurized juices (fruit and vegetable)

Treating Food Poisoning

Having a food-borne illness can be miserable. While you think you might die, most cases are over within a few short hours. If a food-borne illness is not serious and doesn't meet the criteria for seeking medical care, it can be treated at home.

Food Poisoning Self-Care

The most important thing to do is stay hydrated. Drink small sips of clear fluids as often as you can. Water is fine, as are diluted sports drinks. Avoid caffeinated beverages, alcohol, or sugary drinks. Don't start eating until vomiting has stopped. When it has, eat only bland, easy-to-digest foods, like rice, potatoes, low-sugar cereals, and lean meat. You can take an over-the-counter medication for nausea, but never take more than the recommended dose.

Call Your Doctor

If you think you have eaten contaminated food, call your local Poison Control Center. They can answer questions and provide information on what to do next. Poison Control Centers are usually listed with other emergency numbers in your telephone book.

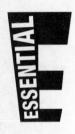

The body uses a large volume of water in the digestive process, and if it loses too much too quickly, severe dehydration can occur. That puts you at risk for other complications, like shock. Be on the lookout for signs of dehydration, which include: pale, clammy skin, crying without tears, and dry, cracked lips.

Children, pregnant women, and people with chronic conditions, such as diabetes or HIV, should contact their physician at any sign of a food-borne illness.

Contact your physician if you:

- Have diarrhea and are unable to drink fluids due to nausea or vomiting
- Are on diuretics and have diarrhea, nausea, or vomiting
- Have diarrhea that lasts for more than two to three days
- Have blood in your stools
- Have a fever over 101°F

Call 911 or take the person to the emergency room if bleeding is excessive or your stools are maroon or black; you are short of breath or having trouble breathing or swallowing; your heart is racing, pounding, or skipping; or you may have poisoning from mushrooms, fish, or from canned food, which might indicate botulism.

When you seek medical care, the physician will want to first assess how sick you are, then determine the cause. The physician will perform a physical, order blood tests, and may do urine and fecal screens. If the illness is caused by a toxin, treatment options may include pumping the stomach or giving medications as antidotes. For a microorganism, rehydrating the patient is often the first concern. Antibiotics are sometimes given, but usually just in cases of travelers' diarrhea.

Common Offenders

There are two main causes of food poisoning: infectious agents and toxic agents. Infectious agents are most common and include viruses, bacteria, and parasites. Toxic agents include poisonous mushrooms, improperly prepared exotic foods (such as barracuda), or pesticides on fruits and vegetables.

Bad Bacteria

Some bacteria infect the intestines, causing inflammation and difficulty absorbing nutrients and water, leading to diarrhea. Other bacteria produce chemicals in foods (known as toxins) that are poisonous to the human digestive system. When eaten, these chemicals can lead to nausea and vomiting, kidney failure, and even death.

Salmonella causes bloody diarrhea in about 40,000 people each year. Ground beef, eggs, improperly pasteurized dairy products, undercooked pork, and poultry products are among the foods linked to salmonella outbreaks. The bacteria *Campylobacter* is also a common culprit in diarrheal illness and can cause symptoms such as diarrhea, cramping, abdominal pain, fever, nausea, and vomiting. About 100 people die annually from salmonella, and it is usually linked back to raw or undercooked poultry meat. In fact, what most people don't realize is that 80 to 100 percent of chickens in the United States carry this bacterium.

Dangerous Viruses

Norovirus and hepatitis A are viruses that have the ability to make you very ill. Hepatitis A can cause you to have a sudden fever, malaise, nausea, anorexia, and abdominal pain. It is usually followed by jaundice several days later. Hepatitis A can be linked back to anything from lunch meat, fruits and fruit juices, milk and milk products, vegetables, salads, shellfish, and even iced drinks. People who are infected with either the norovirus or hepatitis virus and who work in food processing plants and restaurants can pass along the virus. Norovirus outbreaks are commonly linked back to shellfish, like raw clams and oysters, and salad ingredients.

Harmful Toxins

Most people have heard of poisonous mushrooms, and they can be a danger, causing symptoms as mild as a headache or as serious as death. There are other ways toxic food can make you sick. Some large game fish from tropical waters—like barracuda, grouper, snapper, and jacks can all cause ciguatera, a food poisoning produced by a particularly nasty marine algae. Symptoms like nausea, vomiting, muscle pain, and dizziness can last anywhere from a few days to a few years. Pesticides on unwashed produce can cause mild to severe illness with weakness, blurred vision, headache, cramps, diarrhea, increased production of saliva, and shaking of the arms and legs.

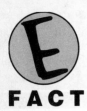

FACT

From the time ancient history has been recorded, parasites like tapeworms have been around. In fact, tapeworms were found in a 3,000-year-old mummy. Early papyrus scripts prescribe using garlic, honey, and vinegar to get rid of them.

Pesky Parasites

Other organisms that can show up in your food and water supply and create havoc are parasites. Parasites are usually defined as organisms that obtain nourishment from another organism, without giving any benefit in return. In most industrialized countries, parasites are rarely a problem, but in developing countries, the problem can be serious.

Parasites usually latch on to the intestine and maintain their nutrition by absorbing partially digested food through the surface of their skin. In other words, they eat the food and nutrients designed for the host. They can cause abdominal discomfort, nervousness, fever, and weight loss.

Food-Borne Illness Diagnosis

Symptoms of a food-borne illness can include gas, bloating, mucus in the stools, chronic fatigue, weakness, insomnia, and itching in the anus or ears. It can be very difficult to get an accurate diagnosis with parasites. Intestinal parasites are often ruled out with a stool sample. A more sensitive test, the Enzyme-Linked ImmunoSorbent Assay or ELISA test, may be ordered. The best testing is done in dedicated parasitology labs, which are few and far between.

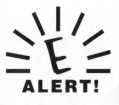
ALERT!

Several different parasites make their home at the zoo and aquarium. Petting zoos are a particularly popular place for bacteria as are aquarium "touch tanks." Don't let little ones touch if you can't clean their hands right away, and make sure you carry hand sanitizer with you in case the facility does not offer any.

More than two thirds of people who are infected may have no signs or symptoms of illness, even though the parasite is living in their intestines. If you suspect you may have a parasite, especially if you have traveled overseas, been to a petting zoo, or you or your child are frequently in a high-contact setting like a nursing home or daycare center, then call your physician.

Preventing Parasites

Watch what you drink. Drink only from water supplies that have been approved by local health authorities. If your water comes from a well, have your water checked on a regular basis. When you go camping or hiking, bring your own water, and don't drink from streams or rivers. Wash raw fruits and vegetables well before you eat them. Wash your hands well before you cook food for yourself or for your family. Encourage your kids to wash their hands after every trip to the bathroom and especially before eating. Kids are inherently unsanitary, but if you can prevent them from eating dirt, it's a good thing.

Be very cautious about eating wild game, as over 60 percent of deer tested positive for at least one type of parasite. Wild animals, ranging from bears to cougars will often eat other wild animals, such as mice that have fed on parasite-infected meat. Take great care about eating any raw or uncooked meat. Uncooked pork, for example, can host a number of different parasites, particularly toxoplasma infection. Undercooked lamb and beef can also cause toxoplasmosis, which can cause serious problems for newborns, the elderly, and those who are already immuno-compromised.

Food Safety at Home

For the average family, about half of your meals will be eaten at home. From the moment it hits your grocery cart until you eat it, you have plenty of opportunities to practice good food safety guidelines.

Buying Food Safely

Food safety begins with selection of food in the grocery store. Your first line of defense is to make sure the store is spotless. It should look and smell clean, especially around the meat, seafood, and produce departments.

Check dates and food labels carefully. As a rule, stores place their freshest foods at the back of the case so the oldest products sell first. There is some confusion about the meaning of the expiration date. It is not a sell-by date, but a warning to consumers not to eat the product after this date. Even if it is marked-down, do not take risks and purchase or consume foods that have an expired use-by date or sell-by date. Check out the packaging as well. Is it tightly sealed? Damaged in any way? For example, all canned foods should have a vacuum seal, as shown by a concave lid. Dented or bulging cans should never be purchased, but should be brought to the attention of the management.

Get in the habit of choosing your meat, poultry, and seafood last. When you are in the produce department, pick up some extra plastic bags and wrap each package of meat in an individual bag. Why? It is the best way to prevent juices from dripping onto other foods. Plus, put your meat at the bottom of the shopping cart, so it is less likely to get in contact with other foods.

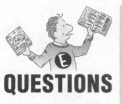

What do I look for when buying fresh fish?
Fish should never have a strong fishy odor. Look for firm flesh, good color, bright, clear eyes and bright gills. If the fish has soft flesh, slimy gills, opaque or dull and sunken eyes and a fishy odor, do not buy it!

Make sure grocery shopping is last on your list of errands. Chilled and frozen foods need to be refrigerated as soon as possible after grocery shopping. Your refrigerator should be set below 40°F, and the freezer should be set at 0°F. A delay in refrigerating can result in multiplying microorganisms.

Preparing Food Safely

The number one contributing factor of food-borne illnesses at home is improper storage and holding temperature of food. Buy an inexpensive thermometer for your freezer (it should be 0°F) and one for your refrigerator (between 40°F and 42°F).

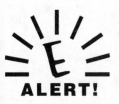

Very few people wash the lettuce and other greens found in the convenient bagged salads from the grocery store. Bags compiled in unsanitary conditions have led to severe food-borne disease incidents, including E. coli. Wash each leaf carefully!

Wash your hands often. Wash hands before, during, and after meal preparation. Proper hand washing may eliminate nearly half of all cases of food-borne illness and significantly reduce the spread of the common cold and flu.

Besides washing your hands, wash all fruits and vegetables. While not often thought of as a source of food-borne illness, fruits and vegetables can easily become contaminated. If produce is irrigated with water containing untreated animal or human waste, if the soil contains pathogens, or if those who pick and handle the produce are infected, then the food is likely to become infected as well. Contaminated produce has caused outbreaks of typhoid fever, cholera, hepatitis, and amebiasis.

When food is cooked to the correct temperatures, harmful bacteria are destroyed. This may sound odd, but get in the habit of reheating hot dogs, luncheon meats (cold cuts), fermented and dry sausage, and all deli-style meat. Heat until steaming hot, even though they are precooked. Why? They can easily become contaminated with harmful organisms after the meat has been processed and packaged.

One of the cheapest and easiest kitchen tools to keep your family safe is a meat thermometer. Generally about $5, a meat thermometer is the only reliable way to tell if your meat is properly cooked. Too often, home cooks rely on the color or texture of the meat to tell if it is done. Hamburger, for example, can be brown, but still not hot enough to destroy bad bacteria. In fact, according to the USDA, 25 percent of hamburger meat turns brown before it reaches an internal temperature safe for human consumption.

USDA Recommended Safe Minimum Internal Temperatures
- Steaks and roasts—145°F
- Fish—145°F
- Pork—160°F
- Ground beef—160°F
- Egg dishes—160°F
- Chicken breasts—165°F
- Whole poultry—165°F

Keep raw meats and ready-to-eat foods separate. Prevent cross-contamination by using two cutting boards: one solely for raw meat, poultry, and seafood, the other for ready-to-eat foods like breads and vegetables. Kitchen stores even sell cutlery boards in different colors to help you remember. If you are going to eat meat within forty-eight hours, it can go in the refrigerator, otherwise throw it in the freezer.

Storing Food Safely

How you store foods is just as important as buying and preparing them. As soon as a meal is finished, leftovers must be refrigerated. Do not stack food containers on top of each other because it limits cooling. Store leftovers in shallow covered containers (two inches deep or less) and consume within three to four days.

Even the way you load your freezer and refrigerator can affect your food safety. Be careful not to overload your freezer or air will not be allowed to circulate evenly. In the refrigerator, keep sensitive items (eggs, mayonnaise, and so on) away from the door panel, because it is the warmest spot. Check your refrigerator at least every two or three days for food that is either moldy or past its prime.

Kitchen Cleanliness

Keeping your kitchen clean really will help keep you healthy. If your counters, cupboards, and refrigerator shelves are wiped down daily with either paper towels and a disinfectant or a sanitizer wipe, it will be easier to keep pathogens at bay.

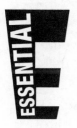

Every two or three weeks, pour a mixture of 1 quart of water with 4 teaspoons bleach down your kitchen sink. Allow it to stand overnight or at least half an hour, then follow with warm water.

If you use a dishwasher, use the heat dry setting. If you wash dishes by hand with soap and warm water, then let them air dry. Don't put dishes, especially silverware, away wet. Never allow dishes to soak in water without adding soap or dish detergent—you don't want to create a microbe breeding frenzy.

Food Safety Away from Home

More than half of all meals are eaten away from home. Since most restaurants carry insurance to protect themselves against food poisoning incidents, you have a responsibility to protect yourself. After all, foods aren't labeled, not all staff have training in hygiene and food safety, and most restaurants aren't inspected by a health department more than twice a year.

Montezuma's Revenge

You want to see the world, broaden your horizons, and meet new people. What you don't want to do is spend your entire vacation locked in the bathroom. Long voyages and jet lag, general fatigue, and change in climates or altitude all reduce travelers' resistance to food-borne disease. The World Health Organization reports that almost half of all international travelers—even those in industrialized countries—will develop some sort of food-borne illness.

Be Prepared

There is no vaccine for traveler's diarrhea. Doctors used to prescribe a dose of antimicrobial agents as a preventative measure, but it also killed off the good bacteria in the gut. Over-the-counter medications like Imodium are also thought to be useless as a preventative measure. In a very few cases, your physician may suggest taking an antibiotic if you are traveling to a part of the world where the food or water supply is deemed very hazardous.

Consuming *E. coliform*-contaminated food or drink is the main cause of travelers' diarrhea, which affects some 27 million adult travelers and 210 million children each year. Travelers' diarrhea usually lasts four to five days, and is associated with nausea, vomiting, abdominal cramps, and dehydration.

Don't Drink the Water

Countries with poor sanitation usually have unsafe drinking water. Water can carry a range of infectious diseases, including cholera, typhoid fever, and dysentery. The other problem with water is that bad water might be used to wash produce and make ice. Keep your mouth closed while you shower and use clean water when you brush your teeth.

Bottled water is a must, but carefully look to see if the cap is properly sealed. Otherwise, unscrupulous sellers can reuse bottles and fill with tap water. If bottled water is not available, look for beverages made with boiled water, such as hot tea or coffee. If you are at sea level, water should be boiled for one minute, and three or four minutes if you are at higher altitudes.

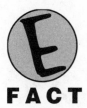

The best prevention of traveler's diarrhea may be information about the country. Your travel agent may be able to help, but the Centers for Disease Control and Prevention (*www.cdc.gov/travel*) offers tips and suggestions on where to look for updated information on the country's food and water supply.

If you can't boil the water, then you will need to chemically treat the water. Chemical disinfectants can be found in large pharmacies. You can add iodine tablets or tincture to water, then let it stand for thirty minutes. Add a squeeze of lemon or lime juice to mask the iodine taste. Bottled carbonated beverages are a very safe bet, especially because it's easy to know if the bottle has been tampered with.

Choose Carefully

While you want to be adventurous in a foreign land, choose where you eat carefully. Hotels and larger restaurants are more likely to be safe, although there is no guarantee. If you choose a small local restaurant or a street vendor, look around carefully. Is the area clean and does the operator cover the food, make it fresh, and keep it hot?

Watch out for seafood, especially if you cannot tell if the fish were harvested close to municipal sewage outlets. Unpasteurized milk and dairy products are associated with increased risk for traveler's diarrhea, so don't just avoid milk, watch out for cheese made from it as well. Raw meat, mushrooms, and shellfish can be risky.

Restaurants Close to Home

Contact your local health department and ask how often they inspect restaurants and how you can gain access to the data. Some departments will publish the information online or in the local newspaper. This information is public, and you should be able to find out how recently a restaurant has been inspected, what violations, if any, were found, and if the problems were remedied.

Be a Detective

When you arrive at a restaurant, look around. It should smell fresh and clean. Are the dishes, tablecloths, cutlery, and any equipment you can see well cared for? Does the staff look as though they care about their appearance? If you are served something that doesn't look, smell, or taste right, do not eat it. Send it back to the kitchen, and do not return. Don't take risks with your family's health.

When you are eating in restaurants, the same rules apply. Don't hesitate to ask specific questions about how the food is prepared. Always request that your food be thoroughly cooked. Don't order meat rare, and if it is served to you rare, send it back. Other potential hazards include raw shellfish, oysters on the half shell, raw clams, sushi, sashimi, and lightly steamed mussels and snails. As you would at home, stay away from any menu items likely to contain raw or undercooked eggs. Common offenders include dressings like hollandaise, homemade mayonnaise, and Caesar salad dressing and desserts such as chocolate mousse, meringue pie, and tiramisu.

ALERT!

Protect your kids at school! Since most kids don't wash their hands before eating lunch, include a hand sanitizer or moist towelette in your child's lunchbox to boost the odds of busting the germs! Teach your children to sing two choruses of "Happy Birthday" or recite the alphabet while they are washing. A regular practice of handwashing for at least twenty seconds will go a long way to encourage lifelong healthy habits.

Chapter 11
Change Your Diet

If you want to be healthy, you must look carefully at the power of healthy foods. Healthy foods have a direct impact on how you feel and on your energy level as well as your longevity and life quality. If you want to live long and avoid disease, there are no guarantees, but researchers are confident proper nutrition is a great insurance policy.

Keep It Natural

By adopting a diet that enhances digestive health, you not only reduce your risk for signs of gastrointestinal discomfort like gas, bloating, and abdominal pain, but you also enhance your overall health. You can start making simple, proactive changes to your diet and lifestyle today that can benefit your digestive health now and all throughout your life.

Eat Seasonally

It is easy to be swayed by special offers, attractive packaging, and ready-to-eat meals. Planning a grocery trip at home can often encourage making healthier choices. Look out for what's new in the produce section. Make it a habit to buy at least one seasonal item every time you shop. Pick some simple dishes using seasonal produce that you can add to your repertoire of meals.

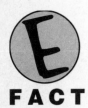

Do you know what's in season this week? Find out what is in season by checking out this website. Updated weekly, use it to discover what's fresh and should be at its best in your grocery store or, better yet, your farmer's market: *www.eattheseasons.com.*

Buy Local

The average mouthful of food travels 1,400 miles from the farm to our plates. Food from local farms is fresher and closer to ripeness, has used less energy for transport, and is less likely to have been treated with postharvest pesticides.

A typical pint of tomatoes at a local farmer's market averages about forty cents more than grocery store tomatoes, but the average time from harvest to market for organic produce is a day, while one to two weeks is the norm for grocery stores. The biggest cost? Grocery store tomatoes lose folate and vitamins A, B, and C due to heat and light exposure.

Avoid Chemicals

Organic farming produces nutrient-rich, fertile soil which nourishes the plants, and it keeps chemicals off the land to protect water quality and wild life. Organic farming also gives us food that is safer to eat and much more likely to keep us healthy. More than 3,000 high-risk toxins routinely present in the U.S. food supply are, by law, excluded from organic food, including: pesticides, metals, and other chemicals.

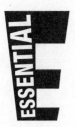

Almost every state has home delivery service of organic produce and groceries. You can set up your order on the computer and within a week, you're set. No order forms. No runs to the supermarket. Just a bag of fresh organic produce, every week, right to your door!

The USDA sets national standards regarding the labeling of organic foods. Organic foods are labeled as belonging to one of four categories:

1. Food that is 100-percent organic may carry the new "USDA organic" label and say "100-percent organic."
2. Food that is at least 95-percent organic may carry the new seal.
3. Food that is at least 70-percent organic will list the organic ingredients on the front of the package.
4. If a product is less than 70-percent organic, the organic ingredients may be listed on the side of the package but cannot say "organic" on the front.

Eating organic produce costs more, but there is a health benefit. More than sixty studies prove that organic produce contains higher levels of some nutrients than conventional fruits and vegetables. Organic crops provide substantially more of several nutrients, including: 27 percent more vitamin C; 21.1 percent more iron; 29.3 percent more magnesium; and 13.6 percent more phosphorus.

Not only is eating organic better for your health, it's also better for the planet. The EPA says that agriculture is responsible for 70 percent of the pollution to the country's rivers and streams caused by chemicals, erosion, and animal waste runoff. It is possible to decrease exposure to pesticides by 90 percent by avoiding those foods that are the most highly contaminated and selecting those that are the least contaminated.

Here are the fruits and vegetables that are highly contaminated with pesticides and therefore you should always buy organic:

- Peaches
- Apples
- Pears
- Winter squash
- Green beans
- Grapes from the United States
- Strawberries
- Raspberries
- Spinach
- Potatoes

Buy Hormone-Free

Many hormones are used by farmers to raise their animals faster and more efficiently. Much of the controversy surrounds beef, since hormones are given to more than 90 percent of cows in the United States.

The use of growth hormones is banned in Europe, and the European Union Scientific Committee for Veterinary Measures has stated that sex hormones used in the United States could pose a risk of cancer and "that children are most at risk."

Eat Fewer Animal Products

Meat and dairy products are major sources of fat in the U.S. diet, and contribute to higher risk of heart disease, cancer, and diabetes.

There's no way around it—too many studies prove the relationship of meat intake to cancer. One study, in fact, tracked two groups, and those with the highest level of meat consumption had increases in the risks of cancer of the colon, lung, esophagus, and liver. The high-intake group did not eat as much meat as you might think—they averaged only one quarter pound of hamburger, or one small steak or pork chop per day.

Choose Minimally Processed and Packaged Foods

About 90 percent of the money that Americans spend on food is used to buy processed foods. Processed foods are foods that come in a box, can, bag, or carton. Generally, the food is far from its original state. Think potato chips, canned soups, crackers, and frozen meals. They are convenient, cheap, and readily available. They are also dangerous for your health.

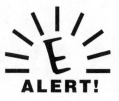

The Food and Drug Administration (FDA) maintains a list of more than 3,000 chemicals used in processed food. These compounds add color, stabilize, texturize, preserve, sweeten, thicken, add flavor, soften, emulsify, and more. But some of these additives have never been tested for safety—they require no government approval. Don't take chances with your health—keep it natural.

As a general rule, the more processed the food, the less nutritious it typically is. Processed foods are typically high in sodium, fat, and artificial ingredients. More important, the more processed foods you eat, the less unprocessed food you eat.

Eliminating processed foods doesn't mean getting rid of every convenience item. Canned, frozen, and juiced fruit and vegetables can be good additions to your shopping cart. When chosen carefully, they are just as nutritious. Buying your fruit and vegetables in this way also means you have plenty at hand when you need it without having to spend time stocking up with fresh produce every few days.

A healthy diet is one with relatively unprocessed foods, including veggies and some fruits and rice or grains that retain some of their original structure to slow digestion. If you look at a processed food and cannot readily identify what it looked like in its original state, rethink it.

Track Your Intake

You will be less hungry if you eat more filling high-fiber carbs as well as a wide variety of good-for-you fruits and vegetables. Not sure what you should be eating? Strive for at least five servings a day of fruits and veggies, but seven or more is ideal. What exactly is a serving of fruit or vegetables? Here are some recommendations:

One Serving Size
- 1 apple, banana, pear, orange, or other similar-sized fruit
- 2 plums, satsumas, kiwi fruit or other similar-sized fruit
- ½ a grapefruit or avocado
- 1 large slice of melon or fresh pineapple
- 3 heaping tablespoons of vegetables or beans
- 3 heaping tablespoons of fruit salad or stewed fruit
- 1 heaping tablespoon of raisins or sultanas (dried seedless white grapes)
- 3 dried apricots
- 1 cup of grapes, cherries, or berries
- 1 dessert bowl of salad
- 1 small glass (150ml) of pure fruit juice

Sample Week Menu for Digestive Health

Following is a sample menu for a week of good digestive health eating.

Day One

Breakfast
Oatmeal—Microwave a bowl of steel-cut oats, add dried plums or seasonal fruit and ground flaxseed. Serve with almond milk or soy milk.

Lunch
Grapefruit Salad—Toss 1 med pink grapefruit (chopped), 2 cups arugula, 1 cup radicchio, 2 tablespoons lemon juice, 2 teaspoons honey, 2 teaspoons

prepared Dijon mustard, 1 tablespoon extra virgin olive oil, and 1 tablespoon coarsely chopped walnuts.

Snack
¼ cup trail mix with dried fruit and yogurt drink.

Dinner
Heat precooked chicken breast strips in a skillet with two cans of diced tomatoes. Season and serve over whole-wheat pasta.

Snack
Low-fat string cheese and seasonal fruit.

Day Two

Breakfast
Two scrambled eggs with low-sodium Canadian bacon and sliced tomato on whole-wheat bagel or English muffin. Serve with blueberry juice.

Lunch
Three Bean Salad—Mix equal amounts of black beans, kidney beans, and chickpeas with chopped red onion and balsamic vinegar to taste.

Snack
Trans fat–free natural peanut butter served on whole-grain spelt crackers and 6 ounces vegetable juice cocktail.

Dinner
Whole grain pilaf with grilled asparagus, zucchini, and bell peppers, with green tea.

Snack
Spreadable cheese on brown rice crackers, fruit, and yogurt.

Day Three

Breakfast

Guava-sauce—Simmer chunks of guava in water until soft, drain and mash. Serve with a whole-grain bagel and yogurt.

Lunch

Spinach salad with walnuts, sunflower seeds, and dried cranberries, drizzled with balsamic vinegar.

Snack

Pretzels and celery sticks with spreadable, reduced-fat cheese.

Dinner

Tacos made with whole-wheat tortillas, ground beef soy alternative, salsa, lettuce, guacamole, low-fat sour cream, and low-fat cheese.

Snack

Yogurt with fresh berries and ground flax seeds sprinkled on top.

Day Four

Breakfast

Cook a packet of plain instant oatmeal, add 2 tablespoons almonds, 1 cup blackberries, and 1 teaspoon honey. Serve with cranberry juice.

Lunch

Turkey breast lunchmeat, bean sprouts, and shredded carrots on whole-wheat bread.

Snack

¼ cup macadamia nuts and fresh fruit or raisins.

Dinner

Grilled trout, baked sweet potato, and coleslaw. To make coleslaw: Mix 1 cup packaged broccoli coleslaw with 1 teaspoon rice wine vinegar and sesame oil. Sprinkle with sesame seeds.

Snack
Whole-grain pita and raw veggies served with hummus, tahini, or edamame (soybean) spread.

Day Five

Breakfast
Toast a whole-wheat English muffin, spread with 2 tablespoons of peanut butter and fruit slices or 2 teaspoons natural fruit preserves. Serve with concord grape juice.

Lunch
Baked potato topped with vegetarian chili.

Snack
Fig bar and fat-free milk.

Dinner
Cook chicken breast strips with 3 tablespoons teriyaki sauce, adding 1 can pineapple chunks. Serve over couscous or brown rice.

Snack
Stir together 1 cup yogurt, 1 tablespoon dill, 3 tablespoons lemon juice, 1 minced garlic glove, and 1 medium cucumber with skin, finely chopped. Chill one hour then serve with crackers or toasted pita bread.

Day Six

Breakfast
1 cup whole-grain cereal with ½ cup fruit and almond or soy milk. Serve with pomegranate juice.

Snack
1 cup mixed melon or seasonal fruit with ½ cup granola.

Lunch

Whole wheat BLT—Two pieces of cooked turkey bacon, sliced avocado, lettuce, and tomato with a thin layer of reduced-fat mayo on whole-wheat bun.

Snack

2 cups honeydew melon with 2 tablespoons flaked coconut and fresh mint.

Dinner

Couscous with mango salsa, grilled turkey or buffalo burger, and salad with arugula and sugar snap peas, dressed with balsamic vinegar.

Day Seven

Breakfast

Black cherry juice, multigrain pancakes (made from mix) with sliced fruit and 1 tablespoon real maple syrup.

Snack

1 cup plum (or other seasonal fruit) spread with 1 ounce low-fat farmer's cheese or other spreadable cheese.

Lunch

Veggie substitute sausage patties, whole-wheat English muffin with cheese slice, and steamed asparagus spears

Snack

¾ cup raw, unsalted almonds and yogurt or kefir.

Dinner

Sautéed shrimp with whole-wheat pasta, pesto sauce, and cherry tomatoes.

Eating Out

It can be difficult to make diet changes because of hectic schedules. A typical fast food meal creates havoc with your digestive system. Keep a collection of quick and easy recipes on hand, so you don't have rely on the same old take-out meals.

Better Fast-Food Options

In the last several years, most fast-food chains have made accommodations for people who wish to make healthier choices. The most popular menu items have the most extra fat, sugar, and salt and are likely to create gastric trouble. Menu items that are fried are going to be high in fat and are likely to create tummy trouble. In sandwiches, wraps, and salads, look for grilled chicken. Choose healthier sides, like a baked potato with broccoli, a fruit salad, or a yogurt parfait instead of oily French fries.

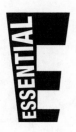

Buy an extra chicken, shred it and freeze it in two-cup portions. In the morning, put your container of chicken in the fridge and it will be ready to use by dinnertime. One rotisserie chicken will give you about four cups of shredded chicken, both white (about 12 ounces) and dark meat with no skin (about 8 ounces).

Eating at Restaurants

Eating late at night can make many digestive problems worse. If it is unavoidable, taking a walk before bedtime may help prevent discomfort. Stick with the basics to avoid the bloated feeling. Here are a few tips to avoid digestive troubles while eating out:

- Request unbuttered buns and toast
- Let the server know that you want steamed, unbuttered vegetables
- Get crackers instead of rolls
- Opt for salads with fat-free or low-fat dressings
- Eat smaller portions

Speedy Dinner Recipes

Simple Chicken Soup

Serves 4

Ingredients

2 cups each of two vegetables of your choice

2 cups shredded rotisserie chicken

2 cans fat-free, low-sodium chicken or vegetable broth

1 teaspoon or less minced garlic

¼ cup or less diced onion

1 tablespoon salt-free Italian seasoning

Soups are a great opportunity to clean out the refrigerator of vegetables that need to be eaten and also a good way to add a wider variety of vegetables to your family's diet. Try diced red potato, celery, carrots, corn, even parsnips, or mushrooms.

1. In a large stockpot, boil vegetables in broth until tender, add chicken.

2. Depending on what you can tolerate, add garlic, onion, and Italian seasoning to flavor.

3. Simmer for 30 minutes and serve.

Rotisserie Chicken Wraps

Serves 4

Ingredients

4 whole-wheat tortillas

2 cups rotisserie chicken, shredded

1 cup diced tomatoes

1 cup shredded carrots

Large handful spinach

Large handful romaine lettuce

½ cup blue cheese or nonfat cheese (if tolerated)

½ cup nonfat salad dressing, or drizzle of olive oil

Wraps are easy, versatile, delicious, and high in fiber.

1. Heat tortillas in nonstick skillet, then remove and cover.

2. Heat chicken in nonstick skillet.

3. Place cooked chicken in center of tortilla, add tomatoes, carrots, spinach, and lettuce leaves. Add cheese and drizzle dressing, then roll the tortilla.

Quesadillas

Quesadillas are a perfect family meal because the heat of the spices can be adjusted to the preferences of each person.

Serves 4

Ingredients
1 red pepper, sliced
1 cup sliced green peppers
    and onions (as tolerated)
4 whole-wheat or corn
    tortillas
1 cup nonfat cheese
2 cups rotisserie chicken,
    shredded
1 cup salsa (as tolerated)
1 cup nonfat sour cream

1. Sauté peppers and onion in nonstick skillet until tender, about 3 to 5 minutes. Remove from skillet.

2. In same skillet, heat tortilla until warm.

3. Onto each tortilla, spoon ¼ of pepper and onion mixture, cheese, and chicken.

4. Fold tortilla in half and cook in a nonstick skillet for 5 minutes, turning once.

5. Serve with sour cream and salsa.

Chicken Fruit Salad

Serves 4

Ingredients

Salad:
3 cups diced roasted chicken breast
½ cup finely diced celery
⅓ cup chopped green onions (the white and part of the green)
1 firm apple, peeled, cored, and diced
⅓ cup dried cherries
1 cup seedless grapes, cut in half
½ cup toasted walnuts

Dressing:
2 tablespoons frozen orange-juice concentrate, thawed (as tolerated)
2 tablespoons creamy peanut butter
2 tablespoons cider vinegar (as tolerated)
2 tablespoons water
1 teaspoon Asian sesame oil

Asian sesame oil derives its dark amber color and nutty flavor from hulled sesame seeds, toasted prior to pressing. It has a strong flavor, so use a gentle hand.

1. Add chicken, celery, green onion, apple, dried cherries, grapes, and walnuts to large serving bowl and toss.

2. Combine dressing ingredients in small jar with tight-fitting lid. Shake well to blend.

3. Spoon dressing over chicken mixture and toss together.

4. You can serve this salad immediately, or you can cover the salad, chill in the refrigerator, and serve the next day.

Sweet Chicken Curry

*Peach preserves make this sweet, and if your dinner guests are
little ones, you can ditch the curry, garlic, and ginger.*

1. Place green beans and carrots in medium glass bowl; cover and micro-wave 6 minutes. Set aside.

2. Heat the oil over medium-high in skillet. Add the onion, garlic, and raisins, and sauté 5 minutes, or until onions are translucent

3. Add chicken broth and peach preserves into skillet and bring to a boil.

4. In small bowl, combine cornstarch with 1 tablespoon water. Whisk cornstarch mixture into skillet, and cook 1 minute. Reduce heat to medium-low, add green beans, carrots, chicken, ginger, and curry powder and heat through, about 3 to 5 minutes.

5. Serve over wild rice.

Serves 4

Ingredients
1 (10-ounce) package frozen green beans
1½ cup carrots, cut into matchsticks
1 tablespoon vegetable oil
1 medium onion, diced (if tolerated)
2 cloves garlic, minced (if tolerated)
¼ cup raisins
1 cup chicken broth
⅓ cup peach preserves
1 tablespoon cornstarch
1 tablespoon water
3–4 cups cooked chicken, shredded
1 teaspoon curry powder
2 teaspoons grated fresh ginger, or 1 teaspoon dried

Chapter 12
Boost Your Fiber

A diet rich in fiber can decrease cancer risks, help you manage your weight, lower your cholesterol levels, and improve your overall health. Since the average diet contains less than 50 percent of the dietary fiber levels needed to be healthy, now is the time to evaluate your diet and learn how and why to boost your fiber intake. Making just a few simple changes in your diet can get you started on the path toward better digestive health!

Dietary Fiber

One indicator of your health is how well you are able to rid your body of waste products. The fiber content of our foods determines how well you do it. Fiber isn't like other food products—it doesn't get digested by your body the way fats, proteins, or carbohydrates do. While those products are broken down and absorbed by your body, fiber passes mostly unchanged through your stomach, small intestine, and then colon.

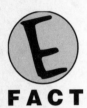

Most people need to double their daily fiber intake. The average American intake is only 10 to 15 grams per day, but the American Dietetic Association recommends 20 to 35 grams each day. Keep a food diary for a week to track how much fiber you're getting.

Fiber Found in Plants

Fiber can only be found in vegetables, fruits, and whole grains. Different plant foods offer different amounts of fiber. To stay healthy, doctors often recommend eating a variety of high-fiber foods.

Types of Fiber

There are two types of dietary fiber, soluble and insoluble. Soluble fiber ferments in the large intestine. It serves to slow digestion and helps your body absorb vital nutrients from foods. Soluble fiber's job is to retain water so that it creates a gel used during digestion. Oat bran, barley, nuts, seeds, beans, lentils, peas, and some fruits and vegetables are all sources of soluble fiber.

The benefits of soluble fiber include:

- It encourages friendly bacteria to grow.
- It helps to control high blood pressure.
- It lowers risk of heart disease.
- It lowers cholesterol.

Insoluble fiber also plays an important role in digestive health. It adds bulk to stool and may help speed food passing through the stomach and intestines. Wheat bran, vegetables, and whole grains are all sources of insoluble fiber. Insoluble fiber helps to:

- Lower risk of bowel disease
- Foster bowel movement regularity
- Keep bowels clean and rid of toxins
- Prevent constipation

Benefits of Dietary Fiber

Dietary fiber increases the weight and size of your stool and softens it. Because it absorbs water, it adds to the bulk. A bulky stool is easier to pass, decreasing your chance of constipation. A high-fiber diet may lower your risk of specific disorders, such as hemorrhoids, irritable bowel syndrome, and the development of small pouches in your colon (diverticular disease).

Fiber May Lower Colon Cancer Risk

Screening for and removing polyps with colonoscopy is the best tool doctors have for preventing colon cancer. Additionally, some research suggests a diet that is low in fat and high in whole grains, fruits, vegetables, and legumes (beans, peas) may reduce the occurrence of some types of cancer, particularly colorectal cancer.

Fiber Lowers Blood Cholesterol Levels

Soluble fiber—found in beans, oats, flaxseed, and barley—binds lipids like cholesterol and carries them out of the body with feces. That process helps lower blood lipid concentrations. In other words, eating whole instead of refined grains substantially lowers total cholesterol, low-density lipoprotein (LDL, or bad) cholesterol, triglycerides, and insulin levels.

Fiber Controls Blood Sugar Levels

Fiber, particularly soluble fiber, can slow the absorption of sugar, which for people with diabetes can help improve blood sugar levels. Some people with mild cases of diabetes given high-fiber diets have been able to reduce their insulin doses. A high-fiber diet may also reduce the risk of developing type-2 diabetes.

Fiber May Aid in Weight Loss

A diet high in fiber can help promote weight loss if high fiber foods replace high-fat foods. In a Tufts University review of several studies, researchers found that women who maintained a 2,000-calorie diet but doubled their fiber intake from 14 grams to 28 grams per day lost an average of four pounds in four months. The best news? Scientists say it can help lose that stubborn belly fat!

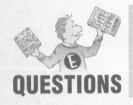

QUESTIONS

Is it true that fiber cancels out calories?
No—fiber doesn't cancel calories, but it can still be considered a dieter's best friend, because it makes you feel full on fewer calories.

The Importance of Whole Grains

Use the U.S. Department of Agriculture's food pyramid as a guide. If you eat two to four servings of fruit, three to five servings of vegetables, and six to eleven servings of cereal and grain foods, as recommended by the pyramid, you should have no trouble getting 25 to 30 grams of fiber a day.

Here are some foods that can help you achieve your quota of daily fiber:

- ¾ cup raisin bran (5 grams)
- 1 red apple (3 grams)
- 2 slices whole-wheat bread (3.2 grams)
- Lettuce and tomato garnish (.5 grams)
- 1 cup air-popped popcorn (1.3 grams)

- 1 cup spinach salad (1.4 grams)
- 1 pear (4.3 grams)
- 1 cup cooked long-grain brown rice (3.3 grams)
- 1 cup cooked carrots (3 grams)
- 1 kiwi fruit (3.1 grams)
- 1 cup cooked oatmeal (4 grams)
- ½ cup navy beans (5.8 grams)
- 1 cup broccoli (5.5 grams)
- 1 cup strawberries (3 grams)
- 1 cup blueberries (4 grams)

The Grain Explained

There are three parts to a whole grain. It is composed of the bran, endosperm, and germ. Refined grains, like white bread or white rice, are made from the endosperm. The bran and germ have most of the vitamins, minerals, and all of the fiber found in grains. Therefore, whole grains are better for you because they have more fiber and nutrients than refined (or processed) grains. Your goal should be at least three servings of whole-grain foods each day.

Besides being a good source of fiber, grains are also good for you because they have many other nutrients, like several B vitamins (thiamin, riboflavin, niacin, and folate) and minerals (iron, magnesium, and selenium). We don't often consider those minerals, but they are critical to being healthy. For example, iron carries oxygen in the blood, and many teenage girls and women in their childbearing years have iron-deficiency anemia.

Another mineral, magnesium, builds bones and releases energy from muscles, while selenium protects cells from oxidation and is necessary for a healthy immune system.

Shopping for Grains

Look for food items that list "whole grain" as the first ingredient and for breads with at least two grams of fiber per serving and cereals with at least five grams of fiber per serving. Less common whole grains include: amaranth, buckwheat, bulgur, kamut, millet, quinoa, spelt, whole-grain cornmeal, and whole rye. "Multigrain" and "stone ground" might be refined and not whole grains.

The Whole Grains Council (WGC) developed the Whole Grain Stamp in an attempt to clarify packaging claims. There are three potential stamps:

- Good Source: at least 8 grams of whole grain per serving
- Excellent Source: 16 grams or more
- 100 Percent Whole Grain/Excellent Source: at least 16 grams and no refined grains. (Sixteen grams equals one full serving of whole grains.)

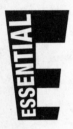

Bored by your bread? Increase the variety of foods you eat by choosing a different bread each week. If you regularly choose a plain whole wheat, then try a rye, multigrain, corn tortillas, or one of the growing number of breads containing seeds.

Here are, according to the Harvard School of Health, some of the more common whole grains for you to look for in your local grocery store:

- Whole-wheat berries are unprocessed kernels of wheat with a nutty, crunchy texture. Look for them in health-food stores or large supermarkets and add them to soups, breads and hot cereal
- Whole-wheat bulgur, whole-wheat couscous, and other strains of wheat such as kamut and spelt
- Brown rice (including quick-cooking brown rice)
- Corn, whole cornmeal, popcorn
- Oat groats, steel-cut oats, rolled oats (including quick cooking and instant oatmeal)
- Whole rye
- Hulled barley (pot, scotch, and pearled barley often have much of their bran removed)
- Triticale (pronounced *tri-ti-KAY-lee*)
- Millet
- Teff (reported to be the world's smallest grain and to have a sweet, malt-like flavor)

- Buckwheat, quinoa (pronounced *keen-wah*), wild rice, and amaranth are considered whole grains even though botanically they are not in the grain family of plants

Tips to Make the Switch

For a change, use brown rice or whole-wheat pasta in place of the same old white flour brand you always buy. It's easy to make the switch and use brown rice stuffing in baked green peppers or tomatoes and whole-wheat macaroni in macaroni and cheese. Then experiment with some new whole-grain products in mixed dishes, such as barley in vegetable soup or stews and bulgur wheat in casserole or stir-fries.

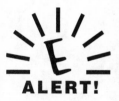

Nutrition facts labels have a glitch—they do not include whether a food's fiber content is intact or isolated. Isolated fiber, which some food manufacturers add to their products, may not have the same nutritional value as natural, intact fiber. To make sure you are meeting your fiber needs, eat 25 to 30 grams a day from whole-food sources such as vegetables, fruit, grains, and nuts.

Adding Fruits and Vegetables

Fruits and vegetables are a good source of fiber. The National Cancer Institute and the United States Department of Agriculture recommend eating five to nine servings of fruits and vegetables each day to maintain optimal health.

Whether fresh, frozen, dried, canned, or 100-percent fruit juice, there are hundreds of ways to add fruit and vegetables to your diet. Experts suggest that up to 90 percent of people do not get enough produce during the day.

How big is a serving? One serving equals:

- ½ cup of fruit
- 1 medium piece of fruit
- ¼ cup of dried fruit

- ¾ cup (6 ounces) of 100-percent fruit or vegetable juice
- 1 cup of leafy vegetables
- ½ cup of cooked or raw vegetables

Eat Your Vegetables

Eating vegetables raw is ideal. It is thought that cooking vegetables may break down fiber into carbohydrates and reduce fiber content. When you cook vegetables, there is no need to cook them until they are soft. Instead, microwave or steam until they are tender. They also have a better flavor. Ready-to-use vegetables are very handy as snacks, quick sides or speedy salads. Just avoid frozen or refrigerated packages with butter or cheese sauces.

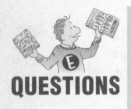

What are some easy ways to boost my veggie intake during the day?
Make veggies as convenient as a box of cookies. Keep a ready stash of dried fruits and vegetable drinks in your cabinets and office. When shopping, look for prewashed, precut vegetables like carrots, broccoli florets, and celery.

Increase Beans and Lentil Intake

Just about everyone can benefit from eating more beans, peas, and lentils. Don't get in the rut of always eating the same kind when there are so many possible varieties on your grocery store shelves. Try black, pinto, or kidney beans; chickpeas; lentils; or (low-fat) refried beans. Add kidney beans to canned soup or a green salad. Another delicious way to boost your bean intake is to make nachos with refried black beans, baked tortilla chips, and salsa.

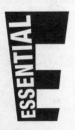

If you like beans, but hesitate to eat them because of embarrassing or uncomfortable side effects, try an enzyme product, such as Beano or Say Yes To Beans, that helps digest complex carbohydrates to prevent annoying "backlash."

Don't Forget the Fruit

An easy way to remember to get more fruit in your diet is to eat fruit at every meal. Apples, bananas, oranges, pears, and berries are good sources of fiber. Try not to peel your fruits and veggies. If you eat the skin and membranes, you're adding extra fiber in your diet. But always rinse with warm water before eating to get rid of any surface dirt and bacteria. When you can, choose whole fruits and vegetables over juice because whole products have more fiber.

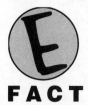

Go slow when adding fiber grams to your diet. Add just a few grams at a time to allow the intestinal tract to adjust; otherwise, abdominal cramps, gas, bloating, and diarrhea or constipation may result.

Fiber Supplements

If you've ever had a bout of constipation, you've probably taken a fiber supplement. Basically, they help to make stool soft, which can ease constipation. Most fiber supplements contain soluble fiber, which means that the fiber absorbs water and forms a gel when mixed with liquid, which is why it can be so useful in helping food move smoothly through the gut. They can be taken as a capsule, chewable tablet, or, most often, as a powder to be spooned into a liquid.

Types of Fiber Supplements

There are several types of fiber used in supplements. The most popular are psyllium, methylcellulose, gum arabic, dextrin, and polycarbophil. Psyllium hydrophilic muciloid absorbs water and expands in the intestines. It is very popular, but can cause bloating and may not be ideal for long-term use.

When you are choosing a fiber supplement, the sheer number of options may feel overwhelming. An important consideration is that the number of grams of soluble fiber varies dramatically from product to product, so don't just look for the cheapest product. Sugar, artificial sweeteners, citric acid, binders, and other added ingredients can give you a dose that is as high as 90 percent filler and only 10 percent soluble fiber.

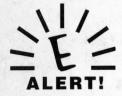

Read the label carefully! If you are sensitive to artificial sweeteners, avoid "sugar-free" versions of fiber. Particularly for many people with IBS, sweeteners like sorbitol, aspartame, and sucralose can upset sensitive stomachs. Citric acid is often added to orange-flavored supplements, and this can cause acid reflux in some people.

It's important to drink an eight-ounce glass of water (and preferably two) with each dose of flaxseed or a fiber supplement. Ironically, both can cause constipation if they're not taken with enough liquid. Whichever supplement you choose, start slowly and gradually increase the amount over time. Don't just stop with supplements, but increase the amount of fruits and vegetables in your diet, eat bran cereal, and do gentle exercise as tolerated.

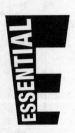

Ask your doctor or a pharmacist whether a fiber supplement may interact with any medications you take. Fiber supplements can decrease the absorption of certain medications such as aspirin, warfarin, and carbamazepine. Fiber supplements can also reduce blood sugar levels, which may require an adjustment in your insulin dosage if you have diabetes.

High-Fiber Recipes

Wheatberry Salad

*Wheatberries store very well unless they are ground. You can cook
a lot up at once and freeze batches for ready use.*

1. Combine the wheatberries, barley, and rice with the water in a medium saucepan.

2. Bring to a boil over high heat.

3. Reduce the heat to low and cover. Simmer until all the water is absorbed, about 1 hour. Remove from the heat.

4. Add the minced onions, garlic (if using), and salt (if desired) to taste. Stir and serve.

Cinnamon Quinoa

*Quinoa isn't a true grain but is the seed from a plant. When cooked, the
germ coils into a small "tail" that lends a pleasant crunch. This is
a nice alternative to oatmeal.*

1. Combine milk, water, and quinoa in a medium saucepan. Bring to a boil over high heat.

2. Reduce heat to medium-low; cover and simmer 15 minutes or until most of the liquid is absorbed.

3. Turn off heat; let stand covered 5 minutes.

4. Stir in fruit, cinnamon, and nutmeg

5. Transfer to four bowls and top with pecans. Drizzle 1 teaspoon honey over each serving.

Warm Vanilla Oatmeal

People who eat more oats are less likely to develop heart disease.

1. Boil water in a small saucepan.

2. Add oats, cinnamon, and salt.

3. Cover and reduce heat to low. Simmer only until liquid is absorbed (about 10 minutes).

4. Add in remaining ingredients, serve warm.

Serves 2

Ingredients
1½ cups water
¾ cup oats (not instant)
¼ teaspoon cinnamon
¼ teaspoon salt
½ cup vanilla soy milk
1 teaspoon vanilla
½ cup chopped dried fruit
½ cup chopped almonds (optional)
1 apple, peeled, cored, and grated

Veggie Stir-Fry

Mushrooms are a good source of the antioxidant mineral selenium, which may offer some protection from prostate cancer.

1. Prepare vegetables by washing and chopping them. Carrots must be sliced into very small pieces or will not cook long enough to be tender.

2. On medium-high heat, sauté garlic, green onion, and ginger in oil.

3. Stir in vegetables, adding water, soy sauce, and mushroom sauce.

4. Let simmer for 1 minute, stirring lightly.

5. Serve warm over whole-grain noodles.

Serves 4

Ingredients
2 cups mixed seasonal vegetables (mushrooms, carrots, broccoli, snow peas)
3 garlic cloves, minced
1 small bunch of green onions, sliced thin
1 tablespoon ginger, sliced finely
2 tablespoons oil
½ cup water
2–3 tablespoons low-salt soy sauce
2 tablespoons vegetarian mushroom sauce (optional)

Broccoli Fruit Salad

Serves 4

Ingredients

6 cups broccoli, lightly
    steamed
¾ cup sweetened dried
    cranberries, raspberries,
    or raisins
½ cup pumpkin seeds or
    sesame seeds (toasted)
1 tablespoon wheat germ
2 tablespoons whole flaxseed
¾ cup light mayonnaise
2 tablespoons raspberry
    vinegar
2 tablespoons granulated
    sugar

One half cup of pumpkin seeds contains 92 percent of your daily value of magnesium, a common deficient mineral. They are also a good source of zinc.

1. In a large bowl place broccoli, dried fruit, pumpkin seeds, wheat germ, and flaxseed.

2. In a small container, mix mayonnaise, vinegar, and sugar.

3. Pour mayonnaise mixture over broccoli mixture. Toss well.

4. Chill before serving.

Rye Cornbread

A single serving of broccoli contains the chemical sulforaphane that kills Helicobacter pylori, *a bacterium that causes stomach ulcers and often fatal stomach cancers.*

1. Preheat oven to 425°F.

2. Mix the first five dry ingredients well. Then add soy milk, Nayonaise, and olive oil.

3. Mix all ingredients together well.

4. Pour mixture into a sprayed 9" × 9" baking pan and bake for 30 minutes.

Serves 6

Ingredients
1 cup yellow cornmeal
1 cup unbleached rye flour
4 teaspoons baking powder
1½ teaspoons sea salt
1½ teaspoons milled flaxseed
    flour
2 cups soy milk
3 tablespoons Nayonaise (as
    an egg substitute) or 2
    eggs
2 tablespoons of olive oil

Easy Bulgur

*Try this as a filling side dish, and experiment by adding different flavors. You can cook it with veggie broth, apple juice, or low-sodium chicken broth.
Each ¾ cup serving has 7 grams of fiber!*

1. Rinse the bulgur and place in plastic or metal bowl, adding salt to taste, but do not exceed ¼ teaspoon of salt.

2. Boil the 2½ cups of water and add it to the rinsed bulgur.

3. Cover and let sit for 25 minutes (if using fine bulgur, let stand 15 minutes), then drain.

4. Toss with the olive oil.

5. Season with basil, salt, and pepper. Serve warm.

Cranberry Pear Sauce

This tastes great served alone or spooned over oatmeal.

1. In a saucepan combine all ingredients.

2. Bring to a simmer over medium heat.

3. Continue cooking for 10 minutes uncovered until cranberry skins pop and mixture starts to thicken.

Fruity Oatmeal Bars

With five grams of fiber per square, these tasty treats sneak some extra fiber into your family's afternoon snack.

1. Preheat oven to 350°F.

2. Mix the oats, cinnamon, flaxseed or wheat germ, and nutmeg in a large bowl. Add dates and apricots, then apple butter. Ingredients should appear moist and well blended.

3. Spoon into a 8" × 13" nonstick or lightly greased pan. Flatten with spatula to make an even bottom layer.

4. Sprinkle brown sugar over surface.

5. Bake for 20 minutes. Remove from oven and cut into 2" squares, then let cool for 20 minutes. Remove from pan when cool.

Serves 18

Ingredients
3 cups quick-cooking oats
1 teaspoon cinnamon
⅓ cup ground flaxseed or
  wheat germ
¼ teaspoon nutmeg
¾ cup dates or prunes,
  chopped
¾ cup dried apricots,
  chopped
1 cup apple butter
1 tablespoon brown sugar

Cheesy Couscous and Veggies

Couscous has 7 grams of fiber per cup and is a mild Mediterranean pasta that complements most meat.

Serves 4

Ingredients

1½ cup unsweetened, organic apple juice

¼ cup water

2 teaspoons olive oil

1 cup couscous

1½ cups frozen peas and carrots

1 teaspoon lemon or orange juice

Pepper to taste

½ cup freshly grated Parmesan cheese

1. Combine juice, water, and oil in a large saucepan; bring to a boil. Stir in couscous and remove from heat. Cover and let sit for 5 minutes while water absorbs.

2. Heat vegetables according to package directions.

3. Add the vegetables, lemon juice, and pepper to the couscous; mix.

4. Sprinkle with cheese and serve.

Chapter 13
Supplement Success

While most people get enough vitamins and minerals to avoid getting sick, it doesn't mean they get enough to stay in peak health. In fact, you are unable to absorb a lot of the nutrients that you take in every day. Food often travels through your system too quickly to be absorbed and used. Anyone interested in living a healthy lifestyle, should research the different recommended vitamins and minerals that can supplement the average lacking American diet.

Consider Dietary Supplements

Our bodies require a lot of different nutrients to function properly. In fact, researchers have identified forty-five known nutrients that are considered essential for good health and must come from sources outside the body. There are at least thirteen kinds of vitamins and twenty kinds of minerals your body requires to function well.

Supplement Benefits

For years, the general wisdom has been that all you need to do to be healthy is to eat a balanced diet and it will provide all the vitamins you need. The catch? No one is exactly sure what the perfect balanced diet looks like. Plus, your unique needs affect what supplements you should take. Someone prone to IBS, for example, may need to take very different supplements than someone with severe heartburn. Your genetics, environment, diet, stress, and health history all play a role in your overall health and what you need to stay healthy.

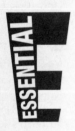

A common mistake people make when adding nutritional supplements to their diet is to go it alone. They self-diagnose health conditions, then create their own supplement plan without once talking to their health care provider. For optimal health, choose a provider whose overall approach you are comfortable with, and talk openly about concerns before taking a supplement, especially when you are combining or substituting them for foods or medicine.

Types of Supplements

Supplements can include vitamins, minerals, herbs, and other dietary substances. Except for a multivitamin, many health care providers suggest taking individual nutrients as separate pills, as opposed to "energy formulas." That way, you can more easily alter the dose of one nutrient without having to change other dosages.

Why would you supplement with vitamins? Dr. Edelberg of WholeHealth Chicago explains, "the fruits and veggies we eat today are less abundant in nutrients than those eaten fifty years ago. In fact, according to research done by Donald Davis, a University of Texas biochemist, they contain from 5 to 35 percent less of some essential minerals and vitamins, like vitamin C, riboflavin, and iron."

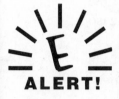

ALERT!

Some vitamins, including vitamin A and niacin, have the potential to cause liver disease when taken in high doses. Others, such as vitamin C and iron, can cause ulcers if they become lodged in the esophagus when swallowed.

Taking Supplements

Usually, unless instructions say otherwise, it is much easier on the digestive system to take supplements with food. Supplements are concentrated, and sometimes they can cause digestive upset or abdominal discomfort when taken in large doses on an empty stomach.

Supplement manufacturers don't have to prove that their supplement is effective the way drug manufacturers do. Instead, they can say that the product addresses a nutrient deficiency, supports health, or reduces the risk of developing a health problem, if that is true. If they make a claim, it must be followed by the statement, "This statement has not been evaluated by the Food and Drug Administration. This product is not intended to diagnose, treat, cure, or prevent any disease."

Choosing a Vitamin

Start with a good multivitamin. Experts say a multivitamin should act as an insurance policy to make sure you get what you need, but real food contains vitamins, minerals, and nutrients that a manufactured vitamin does not. Eating a healthy and varied diet is your best bet.

Beyond the RDA

RDA levels are established by the Food and Nutrition Board of the National Research Council, National Academy of Science. Dr. Edelberg explains, "You need to go above and beyond the so-called recommended daily allowances (RDAs) if you want to effectively use nutritional supplements to prevent disease and slow aging." After all, as one doctor explains, the average American gets most of the RDA of vitamins. However, it is not good to be average—the average American will die early of heart disease, stroke, diabetes, or cancer.

These RDA nutrient levels are supposed to prevent deficiency diseases in most healthy people. Unfortunately, the values are criticized for having been heavily influenced not just by science but also by the food industry, economic considerations, and politics.

Vitamin C

Vitamin C is necessary for a healthy immune system, strong connective tissue, and for general good health. If you are not getting enough vitamin C you may be tired, you may bruise easily, and you may just feel generally ill. Dr. Edelberg explains, "Taking vitamin C is a smart preventive move. It's cheap, safe, and actually works."

Studies show that vitamin C:

- Improves your immune function, both in preventing and fighting infections
- Protects you from developing heart disease, prevents heart attacks, and stabilizes heart rhythm
- Reduces damage caused by high cholesterol
- Reduces frequency of asthma attacks among asthma-prone patients
- Enhances cancer survival
- Promotes healthy bones
- Statistically, can extend lifespan

Dr. Edelberg recommends taking 1,000 to 6,000 mg daily, with 2,000 mg being a good daily dose. The higher doses are generally recommended for people with specific health conditions. The body can not store vitamin C, so daily consumption is important. If you are adding vitamin C with food, do not overcook, as it can remove vitamins.

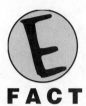

Vitamin C can be completely lost if foods are frozen for longer than two months. Keep your freezer at 0°F to –10°F to minimize this vitamin C loss in juices and vegetables.

Vitamin D

Vitamin D can help protect not only your colon health but also your overall health. A recent article in *Archives of Internal Medicine* showed that people with low levels of vitamin D had a poorer rate of "all cause mortality" than those with levels in the mid-range of normal. Because vitamin D is made in the skin when exposed to sunlight, people living in northern states and Canada are at greater risk of vitamin D deficiency. Specifically, higher intakes of vitamin D (1,000–2,000 IU daily) are shown to decrease the incidence of both colorectal and breast cancer. Besides helping prevent the cancer, another study indicates that patients diagnosed with colon cancer who had abundant vitamin D in their blood were less likely to die during a follow-up period than those who were deficient in the vitamin.

Some sun exposure can be valuable as long as you keep it in a reasonable amount. It may be safer and equally effective to take supplements of natural vitamin D. Natural vitamin D is listed as D3 (or cholecalciferol) on labels. This is not the same as the synthetic D2 (ergocalciferol), which is frequently added to foods or commercial dietary supplements. Your doctor can easily measure your vitamin D level with a simple blood test.

Vitamin A

Vitamin A is another important vitamin for good health. It is known to promote healthy surface linings of the eyes, respiratory, urinary, and intestinal tracts. Why do healthy linings matter? If those linings break down, it becomes that much easier for infection-causing bacteria to enter the body. Vitamin A is also useful to aid the skin and mucous membranes, which function as a barrier to bacteria and viruses.

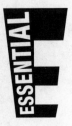

If you are looking for more information on eating healthy, check out *www.fruitsandveggiesmatter.gov*. This website, sponsored by the National Centers for Disease Control and Prevention, has fun tips, recipes, and a feature to help you calculate how many servings of fruits and vegetables you need each day as well as resources for schools and families.

Adults need, on average, about 800 mcg (micrograms) or 5,000 IU of vitamin A per day.

Chronic diarrhea may cause a vitamin A deficiency. A diet that provides five or more servings of fruits and vegetables per day and includes some dark green and leafy vegetables and deep yellow or orange fruits should provide sufficient vitamin A and beta-carotene.

Vitamin A can be found in both animal and plant sources. Animal sources include:

- Pork
- Chicken
- Turkey
- Eggs
- Mozzarella and cheddar cheese
- Egg substitutes

Plant sources of vitamin A include:

- Sweet potatoes
- Carrots
- Broccoli
- Spinach
- Winter squash

- Kale
- Peas
- Sweet red peppers
- Oatmeal
- Tomato juice
- Apricots, fresh and dried
- Peaches
- Apples
- Lemons

Food Supplements

Natural food supplements include many different products—from fish oil to bran and garlic—and are composed of foods that provide a multitude of health benefits. They can be high in certain nutrients, aid in digestion, or offer other benefits.

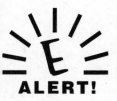

This is one area in which you must be an informed consumer. There are unscrupulous manufacturers who make claims about food products that are not true. Do your own research and talk to a health care provider who is familiar with such products (not all doctors are).

Good supplements come in every form—from jellies to powders to crackers and capsules. Read labels carefully for information on storing and using the products. Their potency may be affected by temperature or shelf life. The book *Prescription for Nutritional Healing* offers a broad overview of food supplements.

Recipes Rich in Vitamins A and C

Western Caesar Salad

Serves 4

Ingredients

1 (10-ounce) package Caesar salad kit

2 cups cubed, cooked chicken breast

1 (14–16 ounce) can low-sodium kidney beans, chick peas, or pinto beans, drained

1 (8-ounce) can low-sodium whole kernel corn, drained

1 medium tomato, diced

1 medium red pepper, thinly sliced

½ medium red onion, thinly sliced

¼ teaspoon cayenne pepper (optional)

One serving of this recipe equals 50 percent of your vitamin A for the day.

1. Mix all ingredients together and top with dressing from salad kit.

2. If you are not sensitive to spices, add the cayenne pepper to dressing before serving.

Cranberry Spinach Salad

Serves 4

Ingredients

1 pound spinach, rinsed and torn into bite-sized pieces

¾ cup pine nuts (toasted at 350°F for 10 minutes)

1 cup dried cranberries or 6 ounces of Craisins

2 tablespoons toasted sesame seeds

1 container of blue or Gorgonzola cheese

¼ cup white sugar

¼ teaspoon paprika

¼ cup white wine vinegar

¼ cup cider vinegar

½ cup olive oil

Limit or change the cheese if you are sensitive to it. The nice thing about using blue cheese is that a little goes a long way.

1. In a large bowl, combine the spinach with the toasted pine nuts and cranberries.

2. In a medium bowl, whisk together the sesame seeds, cheese, sugar, paprika, white wine vinegar, cider vinegar, and olive oil.

3. Toss dressing with spinach mixture just before serving.

Carrots with Pumpkin Seeds

Pumpkin seeds are reported to have many benefits, from improving prostate health to adding phytosterols, compounds that that have been shown to reduce levels of LDL cholesterol. They are also used in some cultures as a natural treatment for tapeworms and other parasites.

1. Peel and cut carrots into 1" pieces.

2. Bring a quart of water to a boil in steamer with a tight-fitting lid. Steam carrots in basket until slightly crunchy, about 8 to 10 minutes.

3. When carrots are done, toss with remaining ingredients.

Serves 4

Ingredients
6 medium-sized carrots
½ tablespoon fresh parsley, chopped
1 tablespoon chopped pumpkin seeds
2 tablespoons lemon juice
1 teaspoon extra virgin olive oil

Kale and Broccoli Stir-Fry

Kale is available year round, but it is best between midwinter and early spring. Rich in calcium, lutein, iron, and vitamins A, C, and K, choose kale with small leaves as it will be more tender and sweet.

1. Heat olive oil in a large skillet over high heat.

2. Stir in garlic and cook for 2 minutes or until golden.

3. Stir in broccoli; cook 1 minute. Add kale and tomatoes, and cook 2 minutes, stirring frequently.

4. Pour in lime juice and soy sauce, and toss well.

Serves 4

Ingredients
⅛ cup extra-virgin olive oil
2 tablespoons minced garlic
1 head fresh broccoli, chopped
2 bunches kale, chopped, with stems removed
¼ cup sun-dried tomatoes, cut in thin strips
2 tablespoons lime juice or raspberry vinegar
1 teaspoon low-sodium soy sauce

Sweet Potatoes and Pears

Sweet potatoes have as much beta carotene as carrots, which may help you fight chronic diseases like cancer and heart disease, as well as diseases related to inflammation, such as asthma and rheumatoid arthritis. Sweet potatoes are also rich in potassium and vitamin C.

1. Place the sweet potatoes in a shallow 3-quart microwave-safe dish; add water.

2. Cover and microwave on high for 18 to 20 minutes or until tender.

3. Drain and place in a large mixing bowl.

4. Add the remaining ingredients; beat until combined.

Serves 8

Ingredients

9 cups cubed, peeled sweet potatoes

4 cups water

4 fresh very ripe pears, microwaved for 2–3 minutes, then peeled

¼ cup packed brown sugar

2 tablespoons butter, softened

¼ teaspoon ground cinnamon

⅛ teaspoon nutmeg

Asian Chicken Salad

Carrots are easily shredded in food processor with a shredding blade. Otherwise, you can shred them by hand or slice thin.

1. Combine cooked chicken with thinly sliced cabbage, shredded carrots, scallions, and almonds.

2. Chop cilantro.

3. Whisk together olive oil, soy sauce, rice vinegar, and honey

4. Toss dressing with chicken mixture. Sprinkle the salad with sesame seeds.

Serves 4

Ingredients

Salad:

2 boneless chicken breasts, cooked and chopped

5 cups Chinese cabbage, sliced thin

½ cup shredded carrot

½ cup minced scallion

½ cup sliced almonds

¼ cup chopped fresh cilantro

2 tablespoons toasted sesame seeds

Dressing:

2 tablespoons extra-virgin olive oil

2 tablespoons soy sauce

¼ cup rice vinegar

3 tablespoons honey

Ginger Papaya Salsa

Eating foods high in vitamin C can help protect cells from free-radical damage, lower your cancer risk, regenerate vitamin E supplies, and improve iron absorption.

1. Combine all ingredients

2. Serve with toasted pita bread.

Serves 2

Ingredients
1 medium papaya, diced
1 tablespoon cilantro, minced
1 teaspoon fresh ginger, grated
1 tablespoon lime juice
½ teaspoon lemon juice

Romaine and Avocado Salad

A cup of sliced raw green bell pepper contains 12 percent of your daily value (DV) for vitamin A, but an equivalent cup of sliced red bell peppers contains 104 percent DV! Red bell peppers provide both color and taste to your meals, along with plenty of both vitamins C and A.

1. To prepare lettuce, remove outer leaves of lettuce heads and discard. Chop remaining inner leaves. Rinse in cold water, dry with paper towels.

2. Tear lettuce into large bowl and add other salad ingredients.

3. Whisk together lemon juice, vinegar, and olive oil in a small bowl.

4. Toss dressing with salad greens.

5. Sprinkle with chopped walnuts if desired.

Serves 4

Ingredients

Salad:
1 large head romaine lettuce
1 large tomato, chopped
1 small red bell pepper, cut in 1" julienne
½ small avocado, cut into chunks
2 tablespoons walnuts or almonds, coarsely chopped
2 tablespoons dried cranberries

Dressing:
2 tablespoons lemon juice
2 teaspoons balsamic vinegar
Extra-virgin olive oil to taste

Peach Meringue

The peaches in this recipe can be replaced with any seasonal fresh fruit.

Serves 4

Ingredients

2 egg whites, room
    temperature
Pinch of cream of tartar
¼ cup sugar
1 teaspoon vanilla extract
3 cups sliced peaches
1 (8-ounce) container vanilla
    or fruit-flavored fat-free
    yogurt

1. Preheat oven to 275°F. Cover a baking sheet with parchment paper or butter it well.

2. Place egg whites into a small, deep bowl. (Metallic bowls will affect egg whites, so use plastic or glass.) Add cream of tartar and beat egg whites with an electric mixer until foamy.

3. Slowly beat sugar into egg whites, 1 tablespoon at a time. Continue beating until stiff and glossy. Add vanilla. Spoon meringue onto baking sheet and spread to a 6" × 9" rectangle.

4. Bake in oven for 1½ hours. Then turn off oven, leaving door closed with the pan inside, for 1 hour. Break meringue, which will now be crisp, into 1-inch pieces.

5. Wash and slice peaches. Layer meringue, peaches, and then yogurt in small bowls and serve.

Cranberry Juice Splash

*One glass of this refreshing drink provides you with more
than 130 percent of your RDA of vitamin C!*

Serves 1

Ingredients

6 ounces cranberry juice
    cocktail
2 ounces orange juice
2 ounces ginger ale or diet
    ginger ale

1. Pour all ingredients into a glass with ice.

2. Garnish with orange slice.

Chapter 14
Ease into Exercise

Eating well is important, and it gives you loads of energy. And once you start to eat more healthfully, you'll probably feel like making other areas of your life healthier as well. Add some exercise into the health equation and you'll quickly feel the benefit. Physical activity combined with a healthy diet will help reduce gastrointestinal problems like stomach pain, diarrhea, and irritable bowel syndrome.

Exercise Boosts Your Overall Health

You know exercise is good for you. Regular exercise makes you stronger and helps you feel better. Regular exercise helps:

- Control your weight
- Reduce physical and mental stress
- Improve digestion
- Sharpen your mental acuity and ability to concentrate
- Strengthen the cardiovascular system
- Lubricate joints
- Strengthen your heart
- Improve mineral uptake in the skeleton
- Lower your cholesterol and triglyceride levels
- Increase your circulation

Besides boosting your overall wellness, a regular fitness program can cut your risks of developing diabetes, breast and colon cancer, osteoporosis, kidney disease, high blood pressure, and arthritis. If you strengthen your immune system, you will be less likely to suffer from other illnesses or disorders.

Exercise Improves Digestive Health

While most people know that exercise offers overall health benefits, most people don't know that it's good for your digestive tract, too. In fact, the World Gastroenterology Organization (WGO) released new digestive health guidelines and included regular exercise as essential.

Regular exercise stimulates intestinal muscles to contract, which causes them to push more food through the system. Even very gentle exercise works the muscles of the bowel, triggering peristalsis (the contractions of the colon that move food along the GI tract) and helps the colon to return to a pattern of normal contractions.

Exercise can help relieve constipation, reduce the risk of colon cancer, and help the body better absorb nutrients. As an added benefit, you may even feel better while you exercise. During exercise, the bowel typically quiets down.

Exercise helps gas pass through the digestive tract quicker, so you feel better faster. Besides relieving digestive problems, exercise can also help prevent obesity, indigestion, and diverticulosis.

And you don't have to be in shape to benefit. One study of 1,801 men and women found obese people who got some form of physical activity were less likely to suffer GI problems than inactive obese people.

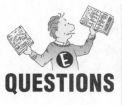

QUESTIONS

If exercise is so important for digestive health, why didn't my doctor suggest it?
Many doctors don't mention lifestyle changes if, in their experience, few of their patients actually make changes, a phenomenon known as poor patient adherence. Doctors do agree that regular exercise is low-risk and helps promote your overall health.

Exercise Helps Your Mental Health

Because exercise is effective in reducing stress, it should also help you with digestive symptoms related to anxiety and tension. When you exercise, your brain releases endorphins, a neurotransmitter sometimes called the "happiness chemical." Endorphins are natural painkillers and antidepressants, so whether you are emotionally hurting or in physical pain, exercise can help. Exercise also helps to balance serotonin, another feel-good hormone. When you exercise you feel better, stronger, healthier, and you have more self-confidence.

Know Your Activity Level

One really useful strategy is to keep an exercise log for a couple of days, similar to a food diary. Write down what you do: how often you walk, how far and how fast, how much time you spend seated—in your job, behind the wheel, or in front of the computer or television—and what physical exercise you get as part of your daily life, such as housework, gardening, or playing with kids.

Add up the total amount of time you spend being active, and the time you spend sitting. Guidelines vary, but you should raise your heartbeat for at least twenty minutes, a minimum of three times per week—these are minimums. Most physicians suggest doing some sort of aerobic exercise for thirty minutes a day; that could mean as little as two brisk fifteen-minute walks daily.

Because exercise helps relieve tension and stress, improves blood circulation, and acts as a mood stabilizer, women who suffer from PMS will also find that exercise helps eliminate or relieve many PMS symptoms.

Getting Started

If you haven't exercised in years, it's always a good idea to check in with your physician first. Most doctors will say as long as you do not have a heart condition, then you go can start moving. Be on the safe side and get a thumb's up before you get up. You may find your health care provider has some good ideas and resources to get you started.

Start Slowly

Starting an exercise routine is never easy, especially if you can't remember the last time you broke a sweat on purpose. Try and get as much physical activity into your life as you can—walking up a flight of stairs instead of taking the elevator, getting off the train or bus one stop early and walking the rest, doing a few simple stretches every day, learning some weight-based exercises, or joining a Pilates class. You have many choices.

As with the healthy eating habits, let your exercise routine develop slowly. Think of one thing you could do regularly to increase the amount of exercise you get. Start doing it. Then add something else, and so on. Encourage your family to join you.

Look for ways to incorporate more physical activity into everything you do. When you go to the doctor, the grocery store, or even the office, park as far away from the door as possible. If you do so every time you park, you can burn an extra 250 calories a day and feel better, too.

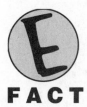

You don't have to make a three-year commitment to the expensive gym to exercise. Many communities have a YMCA (see *www.ymca.net* to locate one near you) or a Jewish community center (check out *www.jcca.org*) that is open to the public and available at a reasonable fee. In fact, some programs offer reduced rates for people on limited incomes.

Start Walking

Walking is the cheapest and easiest form of exercise. All you need to invest in is a good pair of walking shoes. If you are new to any form of exercise, walk for ten minutes at least once a day. After a month, add another five minutes. Keep adding until you can walk for a full half hour. Slowly work toward being able to walk a fifteen-minute mile.

Begin Swimming

It may take a little more effort to find a swimming pool, but swimming is an excellent form of exercise, especially if you have difficulty walking. The buoyancy of the water takes the strain off your body—especially if you have arthritis or suffer pain with weight-bearing exercises.

Listen to Your Body

Many people with GERD find that gentle stretching exercises are the most helpful. Consider activities like swimming, Pilates, yoga, or practicing tai chi. Some people with digestive problems, especially GERD or IBS, may find that rigorous aerobic activities like running or hiking may lead to discomfort. In the same way, some movements, like crunches, may not be comfortable if they force stomach contents into the esophagus.

Take Care

When you have digestive health issues, there are some considerations you need to factor into your exercise plan. Avoid eating two hours before exercise—especially anything fatty or gas-producing. If you do eat before you exercise, pay attention to the portion size. A large meal will require two to three hours of digestion before exercise, while a smaller snack may require only thirty minutes to an hour of digestion. Avoid caffeine or hot drinks before exercising. Both have the potential for speeding up abdominal cramping. Try to time your workouts so you exercise at the times when your intestines are quieter.

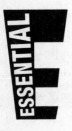

If you are ready to make a commitment to better health, visit your local humane society and adopt a canine companion. Dog owners walk 300 minutes a week on average, while dogless-walkers average just 168 minutes. A human friend works, too.

When you exercise, you may get heartburn when the lower esophageal sphincter (LES) is loose, opens inappropriately, and allows stomach contents to back up into the esophagus. To prevent it, avoid jarring activities like running or jumping and, instead, walk, swim, or ride a bicycle. Drink lots of water while you work out, which should aid in digestion. If heartburn continues to be a problem, you may want to take an antacid before you exercise.

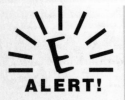

If you have pain in your chest following exertion, you might think it's heartburn when it is angina, or heart pain. Anyone with chest discomfort during or after exercising, even if it feels like heartburn, should be evaluated for heart problems.

Ban Boredom

One of the most common reasons people quit exercising is that it becomes boring. It is easy to get in a rut and do the same walk past the same houses at the same time every single night after dinner. Be intentional about varying your routine from time to time. Choose a different route; even better, corral a friend or your spouse to accompany you. You'll both feel better, and getting some one-on-one time is bound to be good for your relationship, too.

Try Something New

Maybe salsa dancing isn't for you, but Pilates or tai chi might be. How will you know if you don't try? Most fitness facilities will allow you to try a few classes for free or at a reduced rate for a few weeks. Use the opportunity to broaden your horizons. No way you're willing to look like you don't know what you're doing? Then check out the hundreds of exercise videos and DVDs available online and in retail stores. From stretching to kickboxing, you can find the video that's right for your fitness level to do in the privacy of your home.

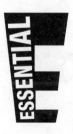

If you have never exercised regularly, getting started can seem overwhelming. Look for ways to incorporate it into your life. Try making it a rule that you can't check your e-mail until you have walked for fifteen minutes. The goal is to weave it into your life as seamlessly as brushing your teeth.

Use this time as an opportunity to try something you have always wanted to do. Want to create a beautiful rose garden? Take up gardening or work on your lawn. Want to be a better mom or grandfather? Get outside and play catch with your child. Need a little extra love in your life? Get a puppy and give it a brisk walk daily. Love watching the reality dance shows? Take dancing lessons and give your partner a spin.

Get a New Attitude

There was a reason you weren't exercising before. You decided it was boring, or you didn't have time, or it wasn't important. For whatever reason, you've changed your mind. Make sure your attitude follows. The mindset with which you approach exercise will play a big role in how successful you are.

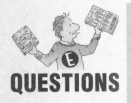

Is it possible to seriously exercise with a digestive disorder?
Absolutely—ask *Vicky Martini, who has had Crohn's, a chronic inflammatory bowel disease for twenty years. She's endured multiple surgeries and had sixteen feet of her small intestine removed. Though the disease creates obstacles in eating and digesting food, it hasn't stopped her from exercising. In fact, she runs half-marathons regularly.*

Exercise is hard, and it's sometimes boring. But with every stretch, every step, every stroke, you are creating a longer, healthier life for yourself. Decide now to approach your workouts with a positive attitude.

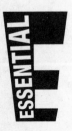

If you are walking, one easy way to set goals is to buy an inexpensive pedometer. Your goals can vary from a certain number of steps per day, or week, or a certain number of steps within thirty minutes, for example.

Set Goals

It feels good to set new goals and reach them. Whether you want to exercise four times a week for thirty minutes a day or walk a mile in fifteen minutes, setting goals can keep you motivated. The only caveat—set goals that are reasonable and attainable. Don't set yourself up to fail. For example, give yourself six months to reach a big goal and celebrate big when you get there.

Reward Yourself

Even if it's a pat on the back, tell yourself what a fantastic job you're doing. Once you can walk a twenty-minute mile, for example, reward yourself with new workout gear or even a pedicure. Be your own best cheerleader! Beginning to exercise is no small feat and every step you take in the right direction is a step toward feeling better and living longer.

Chapter 15
Complementary and Alternative Medicine (CAM)

Alternative or complementary medical approaches are used to refer to non-traditional methods of diagnosing, preventing, or treating pain, disease, or discomfort. Many people, especially those suffering with chronic health conditions like irritable bowel syndrome or Crohn's disease find that these therapies can relieve digestive symptoms or side effects, ease pain, and enhance their lives.

Complementary Treatments

Strictly speaking, complementary medicine is used along with conventional medicine, while alternative medicine is used in place of conventional medicine. This distinction has blurred in recent years as the two groups have begun working more closely together. Doctors now refer to this partnership as "integrative medicine," as chiropractors join orthopedic surgeons, and acupuncturists help pain management specialists. Although a few conventional doctors may still avoid alternative referrals as "voodoo medicine," and a few alternative practitioners warn their patients who value their lives to stay away from doctors, this attitude is quickly disappearing form the American landscape.

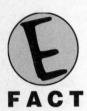

FACT

Children are not small adults. Their bodies can react differently from adults' bodies to medical therapies. In general, complementary therapies have not been well studied in children. Be sure to tell your child's health care providers about any CAM therapy you are considering or using for your child. This helps to ensure coordinated and safe care.

Integrative medicine combines treatments from conventional medicine and complementary medicine for which there is some high-quality evidence of safety and effectiveness. For example, after chemotherapy, a ginger tea may be given to reduce nausea.

Talk to Your Doctor

According to the AARP, more than half of patients over fifty try some form of alternative treatment and do not tell their physician. You may be concerned your physician will disagree with your decision, but you can choose to stand your ground and simply say, "I wanted you to have this information for my charts."

Finding a Provider

The National Center for Complementary and Alternative Medicine suggests asking numerous questions when looking for a provider. Ask about a provider's education and training, their experience in delivering care for your specific condition, and their collaboration with other providers including physicians and licensing (some states have licensing requirements for certain CAM practitioners, such as chiropractors, naturopathic doctors, massage therapists, and acupuncturists).

Whole Medical Systems

Whole medical systems, such as homeopathy, traditional Chinese medicine, and naturopathy, are built upon complete systems of theory and practice. Often, these systems have evolved apart from and earlier than the conventional medical approach used in the United States. While the approach of each system is different, the underlying goals are not directed toward treating a specific illness. Rather, their focus is to bring a diseased body back into balance, empowering the patient to be an active participant in the healing process. These medical systems are very oriented toward overall health maintenance and disease prevention.

Homeopathy

Homeopathy comes from the Greek words for "similar" and "affliction." Its principle is "like cures like"—that substances that cause symptoms of an illness will, in much smaller doses, help the body to heal the illness. Homeopathic medicines are officially recognized by the FDA as over-the-counter drugs and thus any person can order them without a prescription.

Homeopathic remedies are not regulated as closely as prescription medications but even so are considered extremely safe because the active ingredient in a remedy is present in virtually infinitesimally small amounts. In fact, critics of homeopathy point out that the concentration of active substance in virtually all homeopathic remedies is too diluted to have any health benefits. In homeopathic theory, however, the strength of the remedy actually increases when the amount of active ingredient decreases. This concept, which conventional doctors regard as totally unscientific, is the basis for the low regard American medicine holds for homeopathy. Interestingly, homeopathic physicians are well respected elsewhere in the world, especially Europe, the United Kingdom (Queen Elizabeth's physician is a homeopath), India, and South

America. Nevertheless, homeopathic remedies should not replace conventional treatments for serious illnesses.

Colonic Cleansing

Often, many alternative doctors recommend a colon cleansing once or twice each year. A colon cleansing may also be referred to as an "herbal cleansing," "colonic," or "detoxification." According to a *USA Today* article, "Most people who eat the standard American 'goo and glue' diet have about 5 to 10 pounds of matter stored in the colon." Some health care practitioners recommend it to remove toxins from your body and boost your energy and immune systems.

Colon cleansing is critical when you need to prepare for a medical examination of the colon, like a colonoscopy. However, most doctors do not recommend colon cleansing to improve health or prevent disease. The reason behind the concern is that your colon absorbs water and sodium in its effort to regulate your body's fluid and electrolyte balance. The risk in some colon-cleansing programs is that the balance will be disrupted, causing dehydration and electrolyte imbalance. Many physicians insist that if you use a colonic cleansing remedy, you must not use it long term or excessively.

Naturopathic Medicine

Naturopathy seeks to encourage the body's ability to heal itself through changes in lifestyle and diet, as well as herbs, massage, and joint manipulation. Dr. Susan Pilgrim explains that naturopathy focuses on the vital force of life that is inherent in the whole person. When the body is ill, it goes through a self-cleansing process. The underlying conditions that promote the illness must be eliminated. Self-responsibility for health and healing is strongly promoted. However, herbs are considered nutritional supplements and should be discussed with your physician.

Herbs

Many people prefer to take natural supplements over pharmaceutical chemical compounds. Herbal bitters, carminative oils, and herbal teas are just a few of the effective ways to relieve the symptoms associated with digestive disorders. Carminative oils are made from a variety of herbs, usually including caraway, fennel, and peppermint. They are commonly used to relieve indigestion and gas. Herbal bitters refer to individual herbs or a combination; the most well known is Swedish bitters.

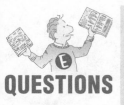

QUESTIONS

I have a bunch of herbs, now what?
Make an infusion. The herbs can be steeped in very hot water, usually for 1 to 3 minutes. Place the herbs in a tea strainer or make your own reusable tea bags out of cheesecloth.

Here are popular herbal remedies for relieving indigestion and bloating:

- One tablespoon of apple cider vinegar taken ten minutes before a meal works as a good digestive aid, especially for fatty food.
- Ginger in cooking, teas, dried powders, essential oils, or capsules works for morning sickness and nausea.
- Aloe vera juice can be helpful for IBS symptoms.

Herbal Tea

Green tea can be very soothing; it is thought to have medicinal properties as well. Green tea consumption is associated with a decreased risk of cancer because of its glutathione s-transferase (GST), a cancer-fighting enzyme produced in the body that helps to detoxify carcinogens.

Why is green tea so good for you? Researchers believe it is due to polyphenols, which are chemicals with potent antioxidant properties. Early evidence suggests the antioxidant effects of polyphenols may even be greater than that of vitamin C. However, it is the polyphenols in green tea that are responsible for its slightly bitter taste.

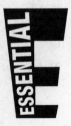

Adding two to three tablespoons of citrus juice (orange, grapefruit, lemon, or lime) to one cup of green tea improves the stability of catechins (antioxidants that help prevent cancer, stroke, and heart disease). Steep one tea bag in hot water three to five minutes, then add the juice.

Try adding lemon or cucumber slices to water for a refreshing twist. Decaffeinated herbal teas are also a great way to hydrate. Following are ten great herbal tea recipes.

Tea Recipes

Ginseng Green Tea

Serves 4

Ingredients
Cold water
Four green tea bags
2 (½-inch) pieces ginseng root
　　(optional)
½ cup honey or to taste

*In Chinese medicine, ginseng is used to reduce stress, increase performance
and energy levels, improve memory, and boost the immune system.*

1. Fill tea kettle with cold water and heat over high until steaming, but not boiling.

2. Place tea bags and ginseng root, if using, into heat-safe pitcher or teapot and pour steaming water over them. Steep for 15 minutes.

3. Remove tea bags and ginseng.

4. Stir in the honey and serve.

Licorice and Fresh Mint Tea

Serves 2

Ingredients
3 leaves fresh peppermint
1 licorice stick, about 1" long
2 cups boiling water

*The licorice stick in this recipe referrers to the root of the licorice
plant, not the candy version.*

1. Pound the licorice stick with a mortar and pestle.

2. Brew in the boiling water with the mint for at least 5 minutes.

Nursing Mom Tea

A good drink for nursing moms with fussy babies.

1. Bring water to a boil, pour over herbs.

2. Steep until water cools, about 10 minutes.

3. Strain and serve.

Serves 4

Ingredients
2 quarts filtered water
2 cups fresh anise leaves
2 cups fresh mint leaves

Peppermint Tea

Peppermint is good for diarrhea, but it is not good for people with heartburn. The leaves are also good brewed with warm milk for those who do not like the tea.

1. Combine boiling water and peppermint leaves. Let the infusion brew for 2 to 5 minutes.

2. Strain and serve.

Serves 2

Ingredients
6 tablespoons fresh
    peppermint leaves,
    crushed
2 cups boiling fresh water

Ginger Tea

Ginger has been used for many years in Chinese medicine. It helps treat stomach pain, diarrhea, and nausea.

1. Peel the gingerroot and slice it into thin diagonal slices.

2. Boil water and add the ginger slices.

3. Simmer for 15 minutes.

4. Strain the tea.

5. Add honey and lemon to taste.

Fennel Tea

Got fresh herbs and the recipe calls for dried? An average guide to use is 3 tablespoons of fresh herb (1 tablespoon of dried herb) for a pot of tea.

1. Use 1 teaspoon of mixture per 1 cup boiling water.

2. Steep 10 minutes.

3. Strain and serve.

Chamomile Clove Blossom Tea

This tea is soothing and is especially good for nausea.

1. Pour boiling water over herbs in a heat-safe pitcher or teapot.

2. Steep 10 minutes.

3. Strain and serve.

Serves 1

Ingredients
1 cup boiling water
½ teaspoon dried gingerroot
½ teaspoon clove blossoms
1 teaspoon chamomile
*   flowers*

Lemongrass Tea

Lemongrass sooths upset stomachs and is good after a heavy meal.

1. Place lemongrass in a heat-safe pitcher or teapot.

2. Pour boiling water over lemongrass and steep for 5 minutes.

3. Serve hot, adding sugar if desired.

Serves 2

Ingredients
2 cups boiling water
3–4 stalks lemongrass, peeled
Sugar to taste

Chai Tea

Serves 3

Ingredients

1 stick cinnamon
¼ teaspoon cardamom seeds
5 whole cloves
½ teaspoon black
    peppercorns
3 teaspoons loose black tea
3 cups water
¼ gingerroot, chopped
Milk, honey, and sugar to
    taste

Good chai is about the color and richness of a good hot chocolate.

1. Lightly crush cardamom seeds and cloves. Mix these spices with cinnamon, peppercorns, and tea and set aside.

2. Add chopped ginger to water and boil for 3 minutes.

3. Remove water from heat and add the tea/spice mixture.

4. Cover and let steep for 8 minutes.

5. Pour mixture through a strainer. Serve with milk and sugar or honey to taste.

What Is Chai?

Chai is a wonderful, spicy tea used commonly in the Middle East to settle the stomach and promote digestion after a meal. Recipes vary tremendously, but it is traditionally made with cardamom and other spices, and stewed or brewed black tea.

Slippery Elm Bark Tea

Serves 1

Ingredients

1 cup water
1 tablespoon slippery elm
    bark (powder)
Milk to taste
Dash of cinnamon,
    nutmeg, or 1 teaspoon
    unsweetened cocoa
    powder, or other
    sweetener of your choice

Slippery elm is very gentle, but great for constipation.

1. Boil the water in a heat-safe pitcher or teapot.

2. Add the slippery elm powder to the boiling water.

3. Add the milk, spices, or sweetener to taste.

Aromatherapy

Aromatherapy is a form of natural treatment that can be used for a large number of conditions. The basic medicine in aromatherapy is essential oil. These oils are extracted from plants and then diluted with almond, evening primrose, or soy oils or alcohol. The oils can be inhaled, sprayed in the air, or applied to the skin. The therapist chooses the most effective essential oil, depending on your condition. There are essential oils for all kinds of conditions, including digestive problems.

The most common essential oils used for digestive problems and their helpful properties are:

- Tea tree oil—fights bacterial fungal infections
- Thyme oil—relieves joint pain and digestive problems
- Black pepper—used for constipation, flatulence, and heartburn
- Chamomile—used for digestive problems and indigestion
- Ginger—used for indigestion

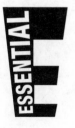

Use your senses—with candles or fresh food, scents like lemon, coriander, sweet orange, and mint are good choices to whet the appetite and get the digestive juices flowing.

A simple and useful aromatherapy blend for digestion uses fennel. Add three drops of fennel essential oil, three drops of lemon essential oil, and three drops of ginger oil to 30 ml of almond base oil. Fennel oil is known to be useful in reducing abdominal pain and trapped gas.

To use as a massage, five drops of the essential oils (concentrated) are mixed with light base oil. To use the oil, massage it into your lower abdomen in a clockwise direction. This follows the natural direction of your colon. Store the remainder of the oil in a dark glass bottle.

To spray the mixture in the air, add ten drops of the oil to seven tablespoons of water, and add one tablespoon of pure alcohol or vodka for preservation. In the bath, add eight drops of oil in a tub full of water and bathe for as long as you wish. A skin patch test should be conducted prior to using an oil that you've never used before. Note: The essential oils are *never* to be taken internally.

Chinese Medicine

In the Chinese tradition, the gentle arts of tai chi and qigong emphasize the lower abdomen as a major reservoir for life energy and health. The belly is considered the "dantian," a key center for higher consciousness development. In Chinese medicine, it is said that negative emotions get processed through the digestive organs the same way food does. Unresolved emotions linger in the organs as an unprocessed charge. When the body accumulates enough unprocessed "garbage," it reaches its breaking point (different for everyone). As a result, the body and digestive health start to deteriorate.

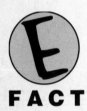

FACT

Traditional Chinese medicine has been used to treat digestive problems for thousands of years. In fact, medical literature dating back to 3 A.D. details specific acupuncture points and herbal formulas for rumbling or gurgling in the intestines.

Acupuncture

According to Chinese medical theory, most digestive disorders are due to disharmony in the spleen and stomach. A study published in the *American Journal of Physiology—Gastrointestinal and Liver* indicates that stimulation of certain acupuncture points inhibits esophageal sphincter relaxations by as much as 40 percent.

Herbal Medicine

There are over 10,000 different natural substances catalogued in the Chinese herbal pharmacy. These substances, known as "herbs," consist of thousands of plant species from all over the world. Mineral and animal materials are often used as well. As a general rule, Chinese herbs are usually taken in a formula, or combination, rather than singly.

Tai Chi

Tai chi, sometimes referred to as an internal martial art, began as a practice for fighting or self-defense, usually without weapons. Over time, people began to use tai chi for health purposes as well. The benefits of tai chi are reported to be massaging the internal organs, aiding the exchange of gases in the lungs, helping the digestive system work better, increasing calmness and awareness, and improving balance. One particular form, tai chi chuan, stimulates the central nervous system, lowers blood pressure, relieves stress, and gently tones muscles without strain. It also enhances digestion, elimination of wastes, and circulation of blood.

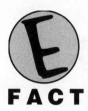

FACT

The art of tai chi is thought to have been created when a monk named Chang-San-Feng back in the thirteenth century was walking through the forest one day. Returning from the Shaolin Temple, he came across a fight between two animals, a crane and a snake. After watching this encounter, he created a set of exercises now known as tai chi chuan, or "meditation in motion."

Manipulative and Body-Based Practices

Manipulative and body-based practices include such practices as chiropractic or osteopathic manipulation and massage. The goal of these approaches is to increase the flow of blood and oxygen to the area being massaged.

Energy Medicine

Energy fields (also called biofields) are a fairly controversial area of alternative medicine, mostly because they have defied clinical proof of existence. Some therapists claim that they can work with this subtle energy, and some patients report benefits, but it is difficult to know if they are simply placebo effects from receiving care from an empathic provider.

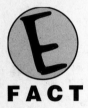

Research indicates that premature babies who were regularly given Reiki, an energy field practice, experienced many positive outcomes. They had better digestion, gained weight faster, had better sleep patterns, performed better on developmental tasks, acquired mental and motor skills earlier, and appeared to be more relaxed than other babies.

Abdominal Massage

Stimulation of your digestive system through an abdominal massage may help your digestive system run more smoothly. Abdominal massage is thought to help improve digestion and relieve irritable bowel syndrome, indigestion, and constipation. You should not eat for two hours prior to an abdominal massage.

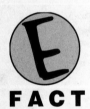

The National Center for Complementary and Alternative Medicine (NCCAM) is the federal government's lead agency for scientific research on complementary and alternative medicine. Besides funding research, they provide fact sheets and educational resources on many forms of alternative medicine that can be found at: *www.nccam.nih.gov*.

Self Massage

If you wish to try this yourself, do an abdominal massage in the mornings and evenings while lying in bed for about fifteen to thirty minutes. With regard to self massage, it is believed that the effectiveness of the massage depends upon the sensitivity to the upward and downward movements (expansion and contraction) of the abdomen. Always work from up the right side and down the left; this is important to aid digestion.

To perform abdominal massage on yourself, begin by placing the heel of your right hand on the right side of the body under the rib cage, and just above the hip bone. As you do so, your fingers should point straight across the body. By pressing firmly, slowly move your hand across your body to the middle of the abdomen. By then, you should have the heel of your hand over your belly button. Repeat this action ten to twenty times for maximum comfort.

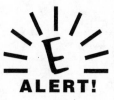

Abdominal massage is not appropriate immediately after abdominal surgery, during an active infection or when cancer is present in pelvic area, while undergoing active treatment of chemotherapy, during pregnancy, or within the first six weeks following a normal vaginal delivery or the first three months after a cesarean section.

Reflexology

Reflexology is a holistic healing art and science performed by a trained reflexologist. The reflexologist applies a sequence of techniques to points found on the feet, hands, and outer ears. These areas correspond to other parts of the body. Pressure is applied with specific thumb, finger, and hand techniques. Unlike massage, it does not use oil or lotion. Trained professionals can use an acupressure chart to find several points relating to the digestion and stomach.

Again, as with other forms of complementary medicine, the clinical data may not be as thorough as for traditional Western approaches. However, clinical reports do show the efficacy of reflexology as a treatment of stress. And anything that relieves your stress is going to be helpful for your digestive system. There is substantial anecdotal evidence that suggests a knowledgeable professional may be able to provide some relief for digestive trouble.

Mind-Body Medicine

Mind-body medicine uses a variety of techniques designed to enhance the mind's capacity to affect bodily function and symptoms. Some techniques that were considered "alternative medicine" in the past have now entered mainstream medicine (for example, patient support groups and cognitive-behavioral therapy). Other mind-body techniques are still considered somewhat alternative, including meditation, prayer, mental healing, and therapies that use creative outlets such as art, music, or dance.

Relax Through Meditation

Usually, a person who is meditating uses certain techniques, such as focusing attention (for example, on a word, an object, or the breath); a specific posture; and an open attitude toward distracting thoughts and emotions. Research shows that regular meditation can lower autonomic nervous system activity. That means meditation allows your body to truly relax. The effect is known as the relaxation response. Not only can meditation and relaxation help you cope better with digestive pain and discomfort, but it will also improve your symptoms.

To begin the practice of meditation, find a place where you can sit quietly without interruption for at least ten to fifteen minutes. A good goal is to work up to twenty minutes. Sit comfortably, close your eyes, and bring your attention to your breathing. As you settle in, silently or quietly repeat your mantra, or phrase of your choosing. For example, "I am healing," "I am well," or "I choose health." You may feel silly, but it is another opportunity to take responsibility for your body and your wellness.

Improve with Hypnotherapy

Unlike any hypnotism show you might have seen, clinical hypnotherapy won't make you lose control, quack like a duck, or do or say anything you wouldn't do normally. Hypnosis is very similar to meditation or visualization, and you don't lose consciousness. Instead, a hypnotherapist will help you relax, and then provide you with suggestions to help your body work in a different way.

Research shows it works. One long-term study with IBS sufferers followed more than 200 people through three months of hypnotherapy sessions. Six years later, 80 percent of the participants reported feeling better for at least five years, saw their doctors less often, and needed less medication than before the hypnotherapy.

The basic premise behind hypnotherapy is that it harnesses the power of the mind to affect the physical symptoms in the body. Researchers have discovered that parts of the brain become more active during a hypnosis session and may direct others parts of the brain to reduce or eliminate their awareness of pain.

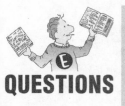

QUESTIONS

How do I find a good hypnotherapist?
The American Society of Clinical Hypnosis is the largest U.S. organization for medical and mental health practitioners using clinical hypnosis. It offers a certification program and can help you locate a practitioner at *www.asch.net*.

Consider Cognitive Therapy

More than 70 percent of IBS patients in one study reported less pain, bloating, and diarrhea after twelve weeks of cognitive-behavioral therapy—a kind of talk therapy that encourages an optimistic frame of mind. It is an active, directive, problem-focused outpatient therapy used for a variety of clinical concerns. Patients meet with a caring, respectful professional who listens to their concerns, helps to define the problems, and assists them in generating solutions and developing better coping mechanisms.

Eat Mindfully

How you eat is just as important as what you eat. There is increasing evidence of a mind-body connection related to our eating behaviors. Surprisingly, when we "tune out" during meals, our digestive process may be 30 percent to 40 percent less effective. And less effective digestion leads to digestive distress such as gas, bloating, and bowel irregularities.

To eat mindfully is to deliberately slow the pace of eating and allow oneself to savor the moment and enjoy the quality of the food. Slow down so you can taste, feel, and smell your food. Following are some ways you can eat mindfully.

- **Sit down when you eat:** At a table, that is—not behind the steering wheel of your car. Do one thing at a time. That means, if you are eating, eat. Don't try to finish your book or send text messages. Closing your eyes while eating can help you to eat mindfully.
- **Don't eat when upset:** Eating when you are upset, sad, angry, or depressed is guaranteed to create problems for yourself.
- **Don't overeat:** Overeating can lead to excess stomach acid, which triggers heartburn. Try to eat small, regular meals. It takes about twenty minutes for the mind to get the message that the stomach is full. Stop eating before you feel full and allow your body to feel satisfaction.
- **Slow down:** Eating too quickly can set off heartburn, so eat slowly.
- **Be quiet after a meal:** Don't jump up to do dishes or the hundred other jobs that absolutely need to be done this very moment. Instead, try to allow yourself just a few moments to sit, enjoy the company (even if it is just you), and be grateful.

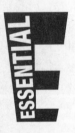

Practice eating mindfully with one piece of chocolate. Break off a small piece of chocolate, then sit down, take a few deep breaths, and look at it closely. Turn it over in your fingers and smell it. Then close your eyes and take a tiny bite—make it last as long as possible. Block out all the distractions around you and concentrate completely on the chocolate. Notice how it feels on your tongue, at the back of your mouth, how it tastes. Enjoy it, savor it.

Chapter 16
Children and Digestive Health

If your child's digestive system isn't working well, her overall health will suffer. At some point, all children have digestive problems, from tummy troubles to constiptation. Learn how to minimize problems and when to get help. The best way to ensure good digestive health is to provide healthful nutrients. If the right nutrients aren't taken in, children may begin to display adverse mental, behavioral, and medical effects. Creating good digestive health starts early.

Children and Good Digestive Health

Poor eating habits don't just cause tummy troubles in little ones. The long-term health risks for a variety of conditions increase as well. Besides setting up your child for a lifetime of poor habits, Dr. Elizabeth Lipski explains in *Digestive Wellness for Children*, "digestive problems are directly linked to a slew of seemingly unrelated juvenile illnesses including arthritis, attention deficit disorders, autism, migraines, asthma, depression, diabetes, and more." Parents and caregivers can recognize digestive factors in children's health and behavioral concerns, find solutions, and encourage healthier habits for the entire family.

Digestive Health Habits

Food allergies, fast food, high-sugar foods, pesticides, and inadequate vitamin intake can create serious problems for children. Poor digestive health habits can lead to digestive health problems such as gas, constipation, and diarrhea. Quite simply, the worse your children eat, the less healthy they will be.

Mood and Learning Problems

Not only does poor nutrition lead to health problems, but it can affect learning as well. Nutritional deficiencies in a child's first years of life, a critical time for brain development, can set the stage for a rough future. According to one study, those deficiencies can cause behavioral problems that can last into the teenage years.

Children with mood and behavior problems may improve if their digestive habits are improved. For example, many parents of autistic children report significant improvements in the behavior of their autistic children after they modify their diet. While eliminating dairy and wheat products for your child's diet may require significant effort, the benefits may well be worth it to attempt it.

If your child has learning or behavioral problems, consider acting as though your child has an unknown food intolerance and begin a food and symptom diary. You may be surprised to see changes in your child's activity level, behavior, or mood when certain foods are either added or eliminated.

Getting Started Right

The best way to protect your children's digestive health may be to breastfeed. Babies who are formula fed are more likely to have sulphurous bacteria in their stomachs. These bacteria are harmful and may cause irritable bowel syndrome later in life. What's more, these infants also have fewer probiotic, or healthy, bacteria, while breastfed babies have high levels of bifidobacter—a bacteria that fights off the bad guys.

Infant Gas

As anyone who ever burped a newborn knows, gas is very common in babies, leading to crankiness and crying. Almost half of all babies suffer from it in their first two months. Infants with gas may try to relieve the symptoms by curling up or pulling up their legs.

Vomiting frequently after eating during the first two years of life means children may have an increased risk of developing heartburn and reflux problems, such as GERD, later in life. Children with reflux problems are likely to have other health problems as well. Potential issues include sinusitis, laryngitis, asthma, pneumonia, and dental problems.

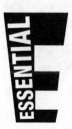

Don't give up if your child refuses a new fruit or veggie. According to the American Academy of Pediatrics, many children will not accept a new food until it has been offered at least ten times. Continue to offer new foods until your child considers them familiar.

Treating Colic

Colic is one of the most common problems during the first three months of an infant's life, and can affect up to 28 percent of newborns. While the exact cause isn't known, some suspect digestive problems may be to blame. Breastfed babies are less likely to develop colic, and there are some studies relating colic to gut flora, especially a lack of *Lactobacillus acidophilus*.

Prevent Food Allergies

Discuss the timing of food introduction with your child's health care provider. Frequently, early exposure may lead to an increased likelihood of problems. Parents are often excited about starting junior on baby food, but may end up creating a food intolerance. Peanut products should not be given until age three at the earliest.

Planning for Good Health

Your child's good digestive health begins at home. From what you buy, prepare, and serve to your family's activity level, you can play a significant role in just how healthy your child is. Almost every family can make improvements in their diet or lifestyle to encourage better eating habits and health.

Buy Organic

One of the best things you can do for your child is to buy organic. If you aren't sure it is worth the money, think again. In terms of relative body weight, children consume more pesticides than adults. The problem is, their bodies aren't prepared to cope with it. Because children's detoxification systems aren't fully developed, they are much more likely to accumulate chemicals over a longer period of time and in greater amounts. Combined with the fact that children are often picky eaters and may only eat a few specific fruits or vegetables, they are more than likely ingesting one particular pesticide or group of pesticides in larger amounts. Unfortunately, this can accumulate to toxic levels rather easily in a small body as chemicals accumulate in muscle or fat tissue.

Aim for a Healthy Weight

In children, being overweight is a significant health concern. Children who have good digestive health will be close to a normal height and weight for their age. Almost 20 percent of children ages two to nineteen are considered overweight. Overweight children are more likely to be overweight teens, who are more likely to be overweight adults.

The health risks associated with child obesity are serious. Children who weigh too much are more likely to develop heart disease, type-2 diabetes, some types of cancer, joint problems, and more. There's also a psychological impact of obesity for kids who don't feel good about their size.

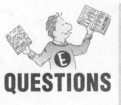

QUESTIONS

What's a fast snack I can keep in the refrigerator for the kids?
Make mini fruit-and-cheese kabobs. Using toothpicks as skewers, thread on fruit and cheese of your choice. You can try pineapple, strawberries, grapes, apples, and chunks of cheddar and mozzarella cheese. Make a big batch and keep in a container kids can reach. If you use apples, dip them in pineapple juice to keep from browning.

Here are some tips for helping your children eat healthy:

- Model good eating yourself.
- Add new healthy recipes to your list of tried and true ones.
- Plan healthy eating for the whole family—for babies and toddlers, teens and adults.
- Make mealtimes a pleasure, and never give food as a reward or withhold food as a punishment.
- Offer a wide range of fresh foods to make sure kids get all the vitamins they need.
- Invite children to help with choosing and cooking food. You'll be giving them a healthy attitude toward food that will last a lifetime.
- Limit fast food.

Limit Sugar

The recommended daily intake of sugar is four to five teaspoons, but many kids consume closer to 25 teaspoons a day. Kids can get 10 teaspoons worth of sugar just from drinking one can of regular soft drink.

No studies show that sugar makes children hyperactive, but it does make blood sugar drop, which could make your children irritable and distracted.

Plus, it contributes to growing obesity rates, leading to higher rates of diabetes, and has other consequences—including tooth decay!

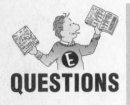

Watch Out for School Lunches

While your child's school may offer healthier lunches, that doesn't mean junior is going to choose them. Often, the same schools that tout healthy alternatives fail to mention that hot dogs, fries, and ice cream are still on the daily menu. Unless your child's school is committed to providing organic, whole-grain foods, start brown-bagging it.

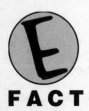

However, that means you will have to be a little creative, so you (and your kids) don't get stuck in the same old PB&J-apple-and-bag-of-chips rut. Put some energy and effort into making it a colorful and flavorful meal. Do not bother with prepackaged lunches. Very few of them are healthy, most are more expensive than what you can prepare on your own, and the excessive packaging is bad for the environment.

When making sandwiches, choose whole-grain slices instead of white bread for sandwiches to boost their intake of fiber and other nutrients. Make it more interesting by rolling it up into a whole-grain pita, wrap, or gyro bread.

Add lettuce, baby spinach, tomato, or cucumber slices to sandwiches to boost their veggie intake. Toss a baggie of baby carrots, sliced cucumber, sweet bell pepper, or celery in the lunch box. Tiny cookie cutters can make for interesting veggie shapes to dip.

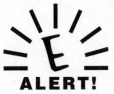

Remember food safety guidelines when packing lunch. Keep it safe by making sure everything is clean, use cold packs for cold items and keep hot foods hot in an insulated bottle stored in an insulated lunch box.

Treats can be tricky. Swap in low-fat cheese cubes and whole grain crackers and swap out the chips to help them bone up on calcium and cut the fat. Fill a sandwich bag with air-popped popcorn for a low-fat, high-fiber snack. Include a baggie of dried cherries with a cup of plain or vanilla yogurt and let them mix up their own sweet treat. Instead of fruit-flavored candy, try dried fruit for a nutrient-packed sweet treat.

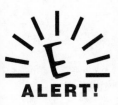

Be careful with choosing vitamins that look like candy. Some look like gummy animals or chewing gum. Make sure whatever vitamins you buy have a childproof lid and are kept out of reaching distance. Accidental overdose of iron-containing products is a leading cause of fatal poisoning in children under six years of age.

Vitamin Power

Ideally, your child should get all of the nutrients he needs from food. According to the American Academy of Pediatrics, a diet based on the Food Guide Pyramid provides adequate amounts of all the vitamins a child needs. There isn't much research on whether adding a multivitamin makes a difference in the health of most children, but there isn't any research to suggest it's a bad thing, either. Many parents prefer to play it safe and think of a multivitamin as a nutritional insurance policy.

If you purchase vitamins, choose a brand formulated specifically for children that provides about 100 percent of the RDA for all of the vitamins and minerals listed. Look for a daily multivitamin with at least 200 IUs of vitamin D if a child:

- Does not get regular exposure to sunlight
- Does not drink at least 17 ounces (500 milliliters) of vitamin D-fortified milk, juice, or soy milk daily
- Follows a vegetarian diet

When Problems Arise

Digestive conditions are often more common during childhood than adulthood. Plus, many digestive diseases start in childhood and progress into adulthood. If the digestive problems are not diagnosed and treated in childhood, there can be long-term health consequences. For example, about 25 percent of individuals diagnosed with IBD are less than twenty years of age.

Children and Diarrhea

At some point, all children get diarrhea. Loose, watery, soft, or more frequent bowel movements are most commonly associated with a stomach virus, especially if it is also accompanied with vomiting and low-grade fever. While uncomfortable, occasional bouts are not dangerous. It usually resolves in a day or two and may be related to a change in diet or anxiety.

Diarrhea can be dangerous in newborns and infants. In small children, severe diarrhea lasting just a day or two can lead to dehydration. Rotavirus is a common virus that can make small children ill very quickly. Because a child can die from dehydration within a few days, the main treatment for diarrhea in children is rehydration.

Call your child's health care provider if any of the following symptoms appear:

- Stools containing blood or pus, or black stools.
- Temperature above 101.4° Fahrenheit.

- No improvement after twenty-four hours.
- Signs of dehydration (dry mouth and tongue, no tears when crying, sunken abdomen, eyes, or cheeks, listlessness or irritability, or skin that does not flatten when pinched and released).

Besides offering plenty of fluids, medication is rarely necessary for children. When your child can eat, your physician may recommend what is called the BRAT diet: bananas, rice, applesauce, and toast. It's very mild and not likely to irritate the stomach.

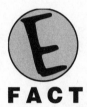

Most cases of diarrhea in children are caused by viruses and will clear up on their own, according to Dr. Joseph Croffie, director of the gastrointestinal motility lab at Riley Hospital for Children in Indianapolis. Parents can ensure their child is getting enough fluids and offer starchy—not fatty—foods, such as dry cereals, oatmeal, bread, crackers, pretzels, mashed potatoes, and rice.

Constipation Tips

Constipation is fairly common among children. Once children are over a year old, many have bowel movements once a day. Almost all children have occasional bouts of constipation. Postponing a toilet trip until after an activity or favorite show may lead to constipation problems later on. Teach her to go when she feels the urge.

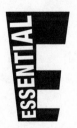

To find a pediatric gastroenterologist near you, go to the website of The Children's Digestive Health and Nutrition Foundation at: *www.naspghan .org/aspModules/PublicLocateDoctor/PublicLocateDoctor.asp.*

Home Treatment for Constipation

Treating constipation in children is similar to treating constipation in adults. Increased fluids, exercise, and a high-fiber diet will all help prevent and treat constipation. Improving those areas will usually be beneficial enough on their own.

Heavy intake of dairy products (even just two to three cups of milk a day) may also create constipation. Soy milk may be a good alternative if that's the case. Sometimes, over-the-counter laxatives may be warranted, but talk to your health care provider first.

Kid-Friendly Recipes

Healthy Chicken Nuggets

Serves 4

Ingredients

1¾ cups herb-seasoned crumb stuffing mix or seasoned bread crumbs

¼ cup grated Parmesan cheese

3 tablespoons margarine, melted

¼ cup low-fat buttermilk or milk

½ teaspoon Mrs. Dash seasoning

4 boneless, skinless chicken breasts (approximately 1 pound)

The chicken nuggets you buy at the grocery store or fast food place are fried in oil, then frozen. These are lightly seasoned, then baked—and taste even better!

1. Preheat oven to 350°F.

2. Pour stuffing mix into plastic zip-top bag. Crush crumbs with rolling pin and add Parmesan cheese. Reseal bag and shake to mix thoroughly.

3. Place melted margarine, buttermilk, and seasoning in medium bowl. Stir well with spoon.

4. Rinse chicken breasts and pat dry, cut each breast into 7 to 8 pieces.

5. Dip each chicken chunk into buttermilk mixture, covering all sides. Let extra buttermilk drip off. Place three dipped chunks at a time into the bag of crumbs. Seal bag tightly and shake until chicken pieces are evenly coated with crumbs.

6. Bake coated nuggets on an ungreased baking sheet for 5 minutes. Flip over then bake other side for another 5 minutes or until brown.

Baked Fish Sticks

This recipe allows you to choose the cuts of fish you would like your child to eat. You don't want to know the kind of fish parts that end up in commercial fish sticks.

1. Preheat oven to 400°F.

2. Put cornflakes into plastic bag and crush with rolling pin.

3. Mix juice into melted butter.

4. Slice fish into 8 pieces. Dip fish pieces into lemon butter mixture, then cover with cornflake crumbs.

5. Place on lightly greased baking sheet and bake 10 minutes, turning once. Pepper to taste.

Pump up the Omega-3s

To slip some more healthy omega-3s into your nuggets, simply mix ground walnuts—a good source of these good fats—into the breadcrumbs. Even if your kids don't like walnuts, they are mild enough that they won't taste them.

Serves 4

Ingredients
2½ cups cornflakes
2 tablespoons lemon juice
2 tablespoons (¼ stick) butter or margarine, melted
¾ pound white fish fillet (such as cod, tilapia, or orange roughy)
¼ teaspoon pepper, or to taste

Perfect Pizza

Serves 1

Ingredients

1 piece whole-wheat pita bread or whole-wheat English muffin

3 tablespoons prepared pizza sauce

¼ green bell pepper

½ teaspoon Italian seasoning

3 tablespoons part-skim mozzarella cheese

If you always thought pizza wasn't a nutritious food, think again. This one has a delicious combination of vitamin-packed peppers, low-fat cheese, and whole-wheat bread. It's great for a quick snack, lunch, or supper.

1. Preheat oven to 400°F.

2. Place bread on baking sheet.

3. Spread pizza sauce evenly on top of bread.

4. Add other toppings as desired.

5. Bake in oven for 8 to 9 minutes.

Orange Peanutty Noodles (for children older than three!)

Serves 4

Ingredients

8 ounces dried whole-grain pasta (spaghetti broken in half)

2 tablespoons smooth natural peanut butter

1 tablespoon orange juice concentrate

1 tablespoon low-sodium soy sauce

1 orange, peeled, cut into bite-sized pieces

You can also add chopped peanuts to the top if your diners won't mind.

1. Cook pasta according to package directions, drain in colander.

2. In saucepan, combine peanut butter, orange juice, and soy sauce; stir over low heat for a minute or two.

3. Remove sauce from heat, add cooked pasta.

4. Add orange pieces; toss and serve.

Easy Banana Treats

A healthy treat for little ones, the texture is very soft and may not appeal to older children. Remember, though, not to give honey to children under two.

1. Preheat oven to 350°F.

2. Mix all ingredients together.

3. Drop by tablespoonfuls onto ungreased baking sheet.

4. Flatten to desired thickness and shape, as cookies will not spread on baking.

5. Bake for 15 minutes then remove to wire rack to cool.

Serves 4

Ingredients
1 cup mashed ripe banana
2 cups oatmeal
½ teaspoon vanilla
¼ cup applesauce (no sugar added)
⅓ cup raisins or dried cranberries, optional
½ teaspoon cinnamon
2 tablespoon honey

Sugar-Free Fruit Sorbet

With high levels of vitamin C and antioxidants, strawberries are a great addition to this sneaky sweet treat.

1. Place all ingredients in a food processor and purée until smooth.

2. Freeze until firm and serve.

Serves 2

Ingredients
½ cup halved strawberries
½ cup raspberries or blueberries
½ teaspoon Stevia Plus (found by sugar on baking aisle)

Breakfast Tacos

Breakfast for dinner is often seen as a special treat, especially if followed by a yogurt parfait.

Serves 3

Ingredients
6 eggs
¼ cup skim milk
Nonfat cooking spray
6 whole-wheat tortillas
Low-fat shredded cheese, for garnish
Low-fat sour cream or yogurt, for garnish
Salsa, for garnish

1. Make scrambled eggs by breaking eggs into a bowl; allow 2 eggs per person. Whisk eggs and milk. Place a nonstick skillet (or regular skillet with cooking spray) over medium heat, and add the eggs. After about two minutes, when the bottom and edges have begun to cook, scrape and lift the edges with a spatula and allow the uncooked part to run under the part lifted. Continue until all eggs are cooked, about 5 minutes.

2. Spoon scrambled eggs into warm whole-wheat tortillas, top with shredded low-fat cheese, a dollop of low-fat yogurt or sour cream, and salsa.

French Toast Sticks

Cutting up this French toast into finger-sized pieces adds to its kid-appeal.

Serves 12

Ingredients
2 cups of egg substitute
Cinnamon, to taste
1 teaspoon vanilla extract
24 slices light whole-wheat bread, cut into strips

1. Combine egg substitute with vanilla and cinnamon to your liking.

2. Dip bread sticks into egg mixture.

3. Cook in a skillet sprayed with nonstick cooking spray for 20 minutes, or until edges are light brown, then flip and cook for another few minutes until light brown.

4. When both sides are brown, eat them plain or top the sticks with sugar-free jelly, sugar-free maple syrup, berries, sliced bananas, or a little powdered sugar.

Sweet Potato Fries

These aren't exactly fast-food French fries, but they are good. Also look for frozen organic sweet potato fries in your grocery store freezer section.

Serves 4

Ingredients
2 tablespoons thawed orange
   juice concentrate
¼ teaspoon sea salt
1 pound sweet potatoes

1. Preheat oven to 400°F and line a baking sheet with foil or spray with baking spray.

2. Cut potatoes into ½" sticks

3. Mix juice concentrate and sea salt in bowl.

4. Dip potato fries in juice mixture, then place on baking sheet.

5. Bake 15 minutes, then flip and cook another 15 minutes.

Whole-Wheat Pretzels

When kids are involved in making their snack, it tastes better. Little ones can practice making letters or numbers. Dip in mustard, cheese, or marinara sauce.

Serves 12

Ingredients
1 cup warm water
1 package yeast (2¼
   teaspoons)
1 tablespoon honey
3 cups white whole-wheat
   flour
1 teaspoon salt
2 tablespoons olive or canola
   oil

1. Preheat oven to 350°F then mix together yeast and water. Let it get foamy.

2. Add in other ingredients and mix well. Add a bit of extra flour, and knead the dough about 20 times. Cover it and let it rise for between 30 minutes and 2 hours. Until it doubles in size. Warm kitchens will get results faster, while cooler, draftier rooms will take longer.

3. Punch dough down, then divide into 12 balls. Make into letters or the traditional pretzel shape, then dip each pretzel in water and sprinkle with coarse salt.

4. Bake about 10 minutes, depending on the size of the pretzels, until golden brown.

Sneaky Pumpkin Waffles

Serves 12

Ingredients
⅔ cup corn meal
1⅓ cups wheat flour
2 eggs
1½ cups low-fat buttermilk
½ cup apple juice or orange
    juice concentrate
1 teaspoon baking soda
1½ teaspoons baking powder
1 teaspoon salt
½ cup canned pumpkin or
    shredded zuchinni
½ teaspoon vanilla

Waffles freeze well. Make them on a weekend morning, then freeze on a baking sheet in a single layer. Toss in a freezer-safe plastic bag or container and you can pop one in the microwave for busy school mornings.

1. Mix all ingredients together.

2. Spray the waffle iron with cooking spray to prevent sticking.

3. Pour batter in the middle of the waffle iron, and spread close to the edge using a rubber spatula. Close the waffle iron.

4. Cook until the waffle stops steaming. Take out and serve.

How can I make boxed pancake mix better for my kids?
Add super-nutritious berries for extra vitamins and healthy plant nutrients. You can also stir some yummy, nutty-tasting ground flaxseed meal (available at any health-food store) into the batter and ramp up the fiber, protein, and omega-3 content.

Sweet Pita Chips

These sweet chips make the best substitute when the kids are craving something sweet. Replace the cinnamon sugar with a little sea salt and they are great for dipping.

1. Preheat oven to 400°F.

2. Spread pita wedges on baking sheet and brush with olive oil.

3. Sprinkle with cinnamon and sugar mixture.

4. Bake for 15 minutes until crisp.

Get Dipping!

Dips are great to get kids to eat more fruits and veggies. Try these types of dips with your kids: ranch dressing, peanut butter, plain or vanilla yogurt, melted cheese, marinara sauce, mild salsa, or tahini.

Serves 4

Ingredients
3 pocket pitas, sliced into wedges and split apart
¼ cup olive oil
¼ cup cinnamon and sugar mixture

Strawberry Pops

Serves 4

___

Ingredients
2 cups frozen strawberries,
    thawed
¼ cup apple juice
2 tablespoons honey
½ lemon, juiced
Pinch salt

You can replace strawberries with blueberries, depending on what is available. Frozen fruit also works, but it may be more difficult to find organic frozen fruit.

1. Combine all ingredients in a blender and blend until smooth.

2. Pour mixture into ice pop molds or ice cube trays.

3. Place in freezer for at least 5 hours or overnight.

Alternative Equipment

If you do not have ice pop molds you can use 3-ounce plastic cups. Pour the pop mix into each cup, cover with foil and insert pop stick through the center of the foil into the cup. Place in freezer for at least five hours or overnight. To remove from the cup, submerge the bottom two-thirds of the cup in hot water for about five seconds.

Creamy Bows and Trees

The creamy sauce will make kids forget they are eating broccoli. Sneak in any other veggies you want, like carrots or julienne zucchini.

1. Cook the pasta according to package directions, drain well, place in a large bowl, and set aside.

2. Cook the broccoli for 3 minutes in a large pot of boiling salted water. Remove the broccoli from the water, and add to the bowl containing the pasta, mix.

3. Meanwhile, in a small pan over medium heat, melt the butter and cream cheese.

4. Pour the cheese mixture over the broccoli and pasta. Toss well.

5. Sprinkle with cheese, if using, and serve.

Serves 4

Ingredients

2 cups broccoli florets

1 pound whole-wheat bow tie pasta

2 tablespoons unsalted butter

1 (8-ounce) package of low- or nonfat organic cream cheese

Freshly grated Parmesan, optional

Appendix A
Soluble and Insoluble Fiber Chart

ITEM	TOTAL(G)	SOLUBLE(G)	INSOLUBLE(G)
Legumes ½ cup			
Chickpeas	6.2	1.3	4.9
Kidney	5.8	2.9	2.9
Navy	5.8	2.2	3.6
Northern	5.6	1.4	4.2
Pinto	7.4	1.9	5.5
Soybeans	5.1	2.3	2.8
Tofu	1.4	0.9	0.6
Cereal Grains ½ cup cooked			
Barley	4.2	0.9	3.3
Bulgar	2.9	0.5	2.4
Couscous	1.3	0.3	1.0
Millet	3.3	0.6	2.7
Rice, brown	1.7	0.1	1.6
Rice, white	2.0	0	.2
Rice, wild	1.5	0.2	1.3
Breads (1 medium slice)			
Multigrain	1.8	0.3	1.5
Pumpernickel	1.5	0.8	0.7
Raisin	1.2	0.3	0.9
Rye	1.5.	0.8	0.7
White	0.7	0.4	0.3

ITEM	TOTAL(G)	SOLUBLE(G)	INSOLUBLE(G)
Breads (1 medium slice)			
Whole wheat	1.9	0.3	1.6
Pita	1.3.	0.7	0.6
Tortilla	1.4	0.4	1.0
Cereal (1 cup)			
Cheerios	2.6	1.2	1.4
Cornflakes	0.7	0	0.7
Raisin Bran	8.4	1.2	7.2
Rice Krispies	0.2	0	0.2
Grits, corn	0.4	0	0.4
Oatmeal	3.8	1.8	2.0
Crackers (1 ounce)			
Butter	0.5	0.3	0.2
Club	0.6	0.4	0.2
Graham, 2"	0.3	0.2	0.1
Ritz	0.5.	0.3	0.2
Saltines	1.2	0.4	0.8
Snacks			
Chips, 1 cup	1.2	0	1.2
Popcorn, 3 cups	2.4	0	2.4
Pretzels, 1 ounce	1.1	0.3	0.8

ITEM	TOTAL(G)	SOLUBLE(G)	INSOLUBLE(G)
Fruits (fresh)			
Apple	5.7	1.5	4.2
Banana	2.8	0.7	2.1
Cherries ½ cup	1.7	0.5	1.2
½ Grapefruit	1.5	1.2	0.3
Grapes, ½ cup	0.8	0.3	0.5
Kiwi	3.1	0.7	2.4
Mango	3.7	1.5	2.2
Orange	4.4	2.6	1.8
Peach	3.2	1.3	1.9
Pear	4.0	2.2	1.8
Prunes, 3	1.9	1.0	0.9
Raisins ¼ cup	1.5	0.4	1.1
Figs, 3	5.3	2.3	3.0
Vegetables ½ cup			
Artichoke	6.5	4.7	1.8
Beets	1.5	0.7	0.8
Broccoli	1.3	0.5	0.8
Carrots, baby	2.8	1.4	1.4
Carrots	1.6	1.1	1.5
Cauliflower	1.3	0.5	0.8

ITEM	TOTAL(G)	SOLUBLE(G)	INSOLUBLE(G)
Vegetables ½ cup			
Celery	1.1	0.4	0.7
Greens	0.4	0.1	0.3
Lettuce 1 cup	0.8	0.1	0.7

Source: Northwestern University Fiber Fact Sheet

Appendix B
Additional Resources

Whole Health Chicago

The Center for Integrative Medicine
Dr. David Edelberg
2522 N Lincoln Ave
Chicago, IL 60614
(773) 296-6700
www.wholehealthchicago.com

American College of Gastroenterology

The American College of Gastroenterology represents more than 10,000 digestive health specialists and is committed to providing accurate, unbiased, and up-to-date health information to patients and the public.
P.O. Box 342260
Bethesda, MD 20827-2260
(301) 263-9000
www.gi.org

The Crohn's and Colitis Foundation of America

386 Park Avenue South
17th Floor
New York, NY 10016
(800) 932-2423
www.ccfa.org

National Heartburn Alliance

(877) 642-2463
www.heartburnalliance.org

International Foundation for Functional Gastrointestinal Disorders

The International Foundation for Functional Gastrointestinal Disorders (IFFGD) is a nonprofit education and research organization that addresses issues surrounding life with functional gastrointestinal (GI) and motility disorders. IFFGD helps improve care by enhancing awareness, educating, and promoting research into treatments and cures for GI disorders. *www.iffgd.org*

Chronic Constipation
http://aboutConstipation.org

Acid Reflux Disease (GERD)
http://aboutgerd.org

Motility Disorders
http://aboutGImotility.org

Irritable Bowel Syndrome (IBS)
http://aboutIBS.org

Incontinence or Urgency
http://aboutIncontinence.org

Digestive Disorders in Kids and Teens
http://aboutKidsGI.org

Digestive Health Research
http://giResearch.org

IBS Self Help and Support Group

www.ibsgroup.org

Irritable Bowel Syndrome Association

www.ibsassociation.org

National Institute of Diabetes and Digestive and Kidney Diseases (NIDDK)

NIDDK, NIH
Building 31, Room 9A06
31 Center Drive, MSC 2560
Bethesda, MD 20892-2560
(301) 496-3583
www2.niddk.nih.gov

American Gastroenterological Association

4930 Del Ray Avenue
Bethesda, MD 20814
(301) 654-2055
www.gastro.org

Nutrition

George Mateljan Foundation

The George Mateljan Foundation is a nonprofit organization dedicated to making the world a healthier place by providing cutting-edge information about why the world's healthiest foods are the key to vibrant health and energy and how you can easily make them a part of your healthy lifestyle.
PO Box 25801
Seattle, Washington 98165
http://whfoods.org

American Dietetic Association

120 South Riverside Plaza, Suite 2000
Chicago, Illinois 60606-6995
800-877-1600
www.eatright.org

Appendix C
Glossary

Acid Reflux

When the lining of the esophagus is exposed to the backward flow (reflux) of stomach acid

Acute

Of short duration (not necessarily severe)

Allergy

An acquired, abnormal immune response to a substance that can cause a broad range of inflammatory reactions

Anus

Lower opening of the rectum

Benign

Noncancerous

Chronic

Continuing for a long time

Celiac Disease

Damage to the intestine of susceptible people by gluten

Colitis

Inflammation of the mucosa (lining) of the colon

Colon

Large intestine

Colonoscopy

Endoscopic inspection of the colon

Colostomy

An opening in the body wall created surgically so the colon can drain

Constipation

Passage of small amounts of hard, dry bowel movements, usually fewer than three times a week

Crohn's Disease

A chronic inflammatory disease affecting any part of the gut

Diarrhea

Loose, watery stools occurring more than three times in one day

Digestion

Breaking down of food to simpler substances for absorption from the digestive system

Enzyme

A protein that speeds up chemical reactions and breaks down food into nutrients that the body can absorb

Esophagus

A continuous tube leading from the back of the mouth to stomach

Fiber

The part of a plant that is not digested and helps to make stools bulky and soft

Functional Disorder

A condition in which an organ does not function perfectly, although it may look structurally normal and the doctor can find no evidence of disease

Gallstones

Stones usually formed from crystals of cholesterol in the gallbladder

Gastritis

Inflammation of the mucosa (lining) of the stomach

GERD

Gastroesophageal reflux disease where the stomach contents regurgitate and back up (reflux) into the esophagus

Gluten

The sticky (glutinous) protein of wheat, rye, barley, and oats

Heartburn

A burning sensation that radiates up from the stomach to the chest and throat

Hemorrhoids

Swelling of blood vessels in the anus. Most often painless, hemorrhoids can become inflamed and painful or can open and bleed

Hiatus Hernia

Protrusion of part of the stomach through the hiatus of the diaphragm

Inflammation

Reddening of a tissue in response to injury or infection

Inflammatory Bowel Disease (IBD)

Disease where the bowel becomes inflamed. Usually refers to ulcerative colitis or Crohn's disease

Irritable Bowel Syndrome (IBS)

A common functional bowel disorder causing abdominal pain, diarrhea or constipation

Polyp

Benign (noncancerous) bowel tumor

Rectum

Lower end of the bowel leading from colon to anus

Index

Cancer (*continued*)

   preventing, 57–74

   risk factors for, 46, 61–62

   screening for, xiv–xv, 63–64

   symptoms of, 63

Carrot Shake, 130

Carrots with Pumpkin Seeds, 205

CAT scan, 117

Cecum, 7

Celiac disease, 76, 79, 83, 139, 272

Chai Tea, 230

Chamomile Clove Blossom Tea, 229

Changes in diet, 159–75

Cheesy Couscous and Veggies, 194

Chicken Fruit Salad, 174

Chicken recipes, 169, 171–75

Chickpea Salad, 73

Children

   and behavioral problems, 240

   and digestive health, 239–59

   and fast food, 243

   fiber for, 244

   and food allergies, 241–42

   and learning problems, 240

   lunches for, 244–45, 250–59

   obesity in, 242–44

   and pesticides, 242

   treats for, 243, 245, 253, 258

   vitamins for, 245–46

Chinese medicine, 232–33

Chiropractic manipulation, 220, 233

Cholesterol levels, 111, 177, 179, 210, 244

Chronic constipation, 14

Chronic diarrhea, 12, 14, 200

Chronic disorders, 12, 14, 200, 272. *See also* Disorders

Cinnamon Quinoa, 188

Cognitive therapy, 237

Colic, 241

Colitis, 44–45, 137, 139, 272

Colon, 7, 272

Colon cancer

   preventing, 57–74

   risk factors for, 46, 61–62

   screening for, xiv–xv, 63–64

   symptoms of, 63

Colon cleansing, 222

Colon habits, 11–13

Colon health, 64–65

Colon health recipes, 67–74

Colonoscopy, 59, 62, 64, 112–15, 222, 273

Colorectal cancer

   preventing, 57–74

   risk factors for, 46, 61–62

   screening for, xiv–xv, 63–64

   symptoms of, 63

Colorectal polyps, 57–59, 98, 114–15, 179, 275

Colostomy, 273

Complementary and alternative medicine (CAM), 219–38

Complete blood count (CBC), 111

Constipation, 39–41, 60, 247–48, 273

Conventional medicine, 220–21

Cooking foods, 154

Cornbread Muffins, 33

Corn Casserole, 90

Craig, Diane, 85

Cranberry Juice Splash, 208

Cranberry Pear Sauce, 192

Cranberry Spinach Salad, 204

Creamy Bows and Trees, 259

Croffie, Joseph, 247

Crohn's disease, 44–45, 137, 139, 216, 273

CT scans, 116, 117

D

Dairy-Free Cake, 94

Dairy-Free Dip, 89

Dairy intolerance, 76, 80–82

Dehydration, 38–39, 121–22, 222, 246–47

Dental health, 9

Detoxification, 222

Diagnostic tests, 109–18

Diarrhea, 12, 14, 38–39, 137, 148, 200, 246–47, 273

Diary, keeping, 12, 15–17, 79, 102, 178, 211

Diet, changing, 159–75

Diet, variety in, 9–10

Dietary fiber

   benefits of, 178–80

   boosting, 177–94

   for children, 244

   supplements, 185–86

   types of, 178–80

THE EVERYTHING SERIES!

BUSINESS & PERSONAL FINANCE

Everything® Accounting Book
Everything® Budgeting Book, 2nd Ed.
Everything® Business Planning Book
Everything® Coaching and Mentoring Book, 2nd Ed.
Everything® Fundraising Book
Everything® Get Out of Debt Book
Everything® Grant Writing Book, 2nd Ed.
Everything® Guide to Buying Foreclosures
Everything® Guide to Fundraising, $15.95
Everything® Guide to Mortgages
Everything® Guide to Personal Finance for Single Mothers
Everything® Home-Based Business Book, 2nd Ed.
Everything® Homebuying Book, 3rd Ed., $15.95
Everything® Homeselling Book, 2nd Ed.
Everything® Human Resource Management Book
Everything® Improve Your Credit Book
Everything® Investing Book, 2nd Ed.
Everything® Landlording Book
Everything® Leadership Book, 2nd Ed.
Everything® Managing People Book, 2nd Ed.
Everything® Negotiating Book
Everything® Online Auctions Book
Everything® Online Business Book
Everything® Personal Finance Book
Everything® Personal Finance in Your 20s & 30s Book, 2nd Ed.
Everything® Personal Finance in Your 40s & 50s Book, $15.95
Everything® Project Management Book, 2nd Ed.
Everything® Real Estate Investing Book
Everything® Retirement Planning Book
Everything® Robert's Rules Book, $7.95
Everything® Selling Book
Everything® Start Your Own Business Book, 2nd Ed.
Everything® Wills & Estate Planning Book

COOKING

Everything® Barbecue Cookbook
Everything® Bartender's Book, 2nd Ed., $9.95
Everything® Calorie Counting Cookbook
Everything® Cheese Book
Everything® Chinese Cookbook
Everything® Classic Recipes Book
Everything® Cocktail Parties & Drinks Book
Everything® College Cookbook
Everything® Cooking for Baby and Toddler Book
Everything® Diabetes Cookbook
Everything® Easy Gourmet Cookbook
Everything® Fondue Cookbook
Everything® Food Allergy Cookbook, $15.95
Everything® Fondue Party Book
Everything® Gluten-Free Cookbook
Everything® Glycemic Index Cookbook
Everything® Grilling Cookbook
Everything® Healthy Cooking for Parties Book, $15.95
Everything® Holiday Cookbook
Everything® Indian Cookbook
Everything® Lactose-Free Cookbook
Everything® Low-Cholesterol Cookbook

Everything® Low-Fat High-Flavor Cookbook, 2nd Ed., $15.95
Everything® Low-Salt Cookbook
Everything® Meals for a Month Cookbook
Everything® Meals on a Budget Cookbook
Everything® Mediterranean Cookbook
Everything® Mexican Cookbook
Everything® No Trans Fat Cookbook
Everything® One-Pot Cookbook, 2nd Ed., $15.95
Everything® Organic Cooking for Baby & Toddler Book, $15.95
Everything® Pizza Cookbook
Everything® Quick Meals Cookbook, 2nd Ed., $15.95
Everything® Slow Cooker Cookbook
Everything® Slow Cooking for a Crowd Cookbook
Everything® Soup Cookbook
Everything® Stir-Fry Cookbook
Everything® Sugar-Free Cookbook
Everything® Tapas and Small Plates Cookbook
Everything® Tex-Mex Cookbook
Everything® Thai Cookbook
Everything® Vegetarian Cookbook
Everything® Whole-Grain, High-Fiber Cookbook
Everything® Wild Game Cookbook
Everything® Wine Book, 2nd Ed.

GAMES

Everything® 15-Minute Sudoku Book, $9.95
Everything® 30-Minute Sudoku Book, $9.95
Everything® Bible Crosswords Book, $9.95
Everything® Blackjack Strategy Book
Everything® Brain Strain Book, $9.95
Everything® Bridge Book
Everything® Card Games Book
Everything® Card Tricks Book, $9.95
Everything® Casino Gambling Book, 2nd Ed.
Everything® Chess Basics Book
Everything® Christmas Crosswords Book, $9.95
Everything® Craps Strategy Book
Everything® Crossword and Puzzle Book
Everything® Crosswords and Puzzles for Quote Lovers Book, $9.95
Everything® Crossword Challenge Book
Everything® Crosswords for the Beach Book, $9.95
Everything® Cryptic Crosswords Book, $9.95
Everything® Cryptograms Book, $9.95
Everything® Easy Crosswords Book
Everything® Easy Kakuro Book, $9.95
Everything® Easy Large-Print Crosswords Book
Everything® Games Book, 2nd Ed.
Everything® Giant Book of Crosswords
Everything® Giant Sudoku Book, $9.95
Everything® Giant Word Search Book
Everything® Kakuro Challenge Book, $9.95
Everything® Large-Print Crossword Challenge Book
Everything® Large-Print Crosswords Book
Everything® Large-Print Travel Crosswords Book
Everything® Lateral Thinking Puzzles Book, $9.95
Everything® Literary Crosswords Book, $9.95
Everything® Mazes Book
Everything® Memory Booster Puzzles Book, $9.95

Everything® Movie Crosswords Book, $9.95
Everything® Music Crosswords Book, $9.95
Everything® Online Poker Book
Everything® Pencil Puzzles Book, $9.95
Everything® Poker Strategy Book
Everything® Pool & Billiards Book
Everything® Puzzles for Commuters Book, $9.95
Everything® Puzzles for Dog Lovers Book, $9.95
Everything® Sports Crosswords Book, $9.95
Everything® Test Your IQ Book, $9.95
Everything® Texas Hold 'Em Book, $9.95
Everything® Travel Crosswords Book, $9.95
Everything® Travel Mazes Book, $9.95
Everything® Travel Word Search Book, $9.95
Everything® TV Crosswords Book, $9.95
Everything® Word Games Challenge Book
Everything® Word Scramble Book
Everything® Word Search Book

HEALTH

Everything® Alzheimer's Book
Everything® Diabetes Book
Everything® First Aid Book, $9.95
Everything® Green Living Book
Everything® Health Guide to Addiction and Recovery
Everything® Health Guide to Adult Bipolar Disorder
Everything® Health Guide to Arthritis
Everything® Health Guide to Controlling Anxiety
Everything® Health Guide to Depression
Everything® Health Guide to Diabetes, 2nd Ed.
Everything® Health Guide to Fibromyalgia
Everything® Health Guide to Menopause, 2nd Ed.
Everything® Health Guide to Migraines
Everything® Health Guide to Multiple Sclerosis
Everything® Health Guide to OCD
Everything® Health Guide to PMS
Everything® Health Guide to Postpartum Care
Everything® Health Guide to Thyroid Disease
Everything® Hypnosis Book
Everything® Low Cholesterol Book
Everything® Menopause Book
Everything® Nutrition Book
Everything® Reflexology Book
Everything® Stress Management Book
Everything® Superfoods Book, $15.95

HISTORY

Everything® American Government Book
Everything® American History Book, 2nd Ed.
Everything® American Revolution Book, $15.95
Everything® Civil War Book
Everything® Freemasons Book
Everything® Irish History & Heritage Book
Everything® World War II Book, 2nd Ed.

HOBBIES

Everything® Candlemaking Book
Everything® Cartooning Book
Everything® Coin Collecting Book
Everything® Digital Photography Book, 2nd Ed.

Everything® Drawing Book
Everything® Family Tree Book, 2nd Ed.
Everything® Guide to Online Genealogy, $15.95
Everything® Knitting Book
Everything® Knots Book
Everything® Photography Book
Everything® Quilting Book
Everything® Sewing Book
Everything® Soapmaking Book, 2nd Ed.
Everything® Woodworking Book

HOME IMPROVEMENT

Everything® Feng Shui Book
Everything® Feng Shui Decluttering Book, $9.95
Everything® Fix-It Book
Everything® Green Living Book
Everything® Home Decorating Book
Everything® Home Storage Solutions Book
Everything® Homebuilding Book
Everything® Organize Your Home Book, 2nd Ed.

KIDS' BOOKS

All titles are $7.95
Everything® Fairy Tales Book, $14.95
Everything® Kids' Animal Puzzle & Activity Book
Everything® Kids' Astronomy Book
Everything® Kids' Baseball Book, 5th Ed.
Everything® Kids' Bible Trivia Book
Everything® Kids' Bugs Book
Everything® Kids' Cars and Trucks Puzzle and Activity Book
Everything® Kids' Christmas Puzzle & Activity Book
Everything® Kids' Connect the Dots
    Puzzle and Activity Book
Everything® Kids' Cookbook, 2nd Ed.
Everything® Kids' Crazy Puzzles Book
Everything® Kids' Dinosaurs Book
Everything® Kids' Dragons Puzzle and Activity Book
Everything® Kids' Environment Book $7.95
Everything® Kids' Fairies Puzzle and Activity Book
Everything® Kids' First Spanish Puzzle and Activity Book
Everything® Kids' Football Book
Everything® Kids' Geography Book
Everything® Kids' Gross Cookbook
Everything® Kids' Gross Hidden Pictures Book
Everything® Kids' Gross Jokes Book
Everything® Kids' Gross Mazes Book
Everything® Kids' Gross Puzzle & Activity Book
Everything® Kids' Halloween Puzzle & Activity Book
Everything® Kids' Hanukkah Puzzle and Activity Book
Everything® Kids' Hidden Pictures Book
Everything® Kids' Horses Book
Everything® Kids' Joke Book
Everything® Kids' Knock Knock Book
Everything® Kids' Learning French Book
Everything® Kids' Learning Spanish Book
Everything® Kids' Magical Science Experiments Book
Everything® Kids' Math Puzzles Book
Everything® Kids' Mazes Book
Everything® Kids' Money Book, 2nd Ed.
Everything® Kids' Mummies, Pharaoh's, and Pyramids
    Puzzle and Activity Book
Everything® Kids' Nature Book
Everything® Kids' Pirates Puzzle and Activity Book
Everything® Kids' Presidents Book
Everything® Kids' Princess Puzzle and Activity Book
Everything® Kids' Puzzle Book

Everything® Kids' Racecars Puzzle and Activity Book
Everything® Kids' Riddles & Brain Teasers Book
Everything® Kids' Science Experiments Book
Everything® Kids' Sharks Book
Everything® Kids' Soccer Book
Everything® Kids' Spelling Book
Everything® Kids' Spies Puzzle and Activity Book
Everything® Kids' States Book
Everything® Kids' Travel Activity Book
Everything® Kids' Word Search Puzzle and Activity Book

LANGUAGE

Everything® Conversational Japanese Book with CD, $19.95
Everything® French Grammar Book
Everything® French Phrase Book, $9.95
Everything® French Verb Book, $9.95
Everything® German Phrase Book, $9.95
Everything® German Practice Book with CD, $19.95
Everything® Inglés Book
Everything® Intermediate Spanish Book with CD, $19.95
Everything® Italian Phrase Book, $9.95
Everything® Italian Practice Book with CD, $19.95
Everything® Learning Brazilian Portuguese Book with CD, $19.95
Everything® Learning French Book with CD, 2nd Ed., $19.95
Everything® Learning German Book
Everything® Learning Italian Book
Everything® Learning Latin Book
Everything® Learning Russian Book with CD, $19.95
Everything® Learning Spanish Book
Everything® Learning Spanish Book with CD, 2nd Ed., $19.95
Everything® Russian Practice Book with CD, $19.95
Everything® Sign Language Book, $15.95
Everything® Spanish Grammar Book
Everything® Spanish Phrase Book, $9.95
Everything® Spanish Practice Book with CD, $19.95
Everything® Spanish Verb Book, $9.95
Everything® Speaking Mandarin Chinese Book with CD, $19.95

MUSIC

Everything® Bass Guitar Book with CD, $19.95
Everything® Drums Book with CD, $19.95
Everything® Guitar Book with CD, 2nd Ed., $19.95
Everything® Guitar Chords Book with CD, $19.95
Everything® Guitar Scales Book with CD, $19.95
Everything® Harmonica Book with CD, $15.95
Everything® Home Recording Book
Everything® Music Theory Book with CD, $19.95
Everything® Reading Music Book with CD, $19.95
Everything® Rock & Blues Guitar Book with CD, $19.95
Everything® Rock & Blues Piano Book with CD, $19.95
Everything® Rock Drums Book with CD, $19.95
Everything® Singing Book with CD, $19.95
Everything® Songwriting Book

NEW AGE

Everything® Astrology Book, 2nd Ed.
Everything® Birthday Personology Book
Everything® Celtic Wisdom Book, $15.95
Everything® Dreams Book, 2nd Ed.
Everything® Law of Attraction Book, $15.95
Everything® Love Signs Book, $9.95
Everything® Love Spells Book, $9.95
Everything® Palmistry Book
Everything® Psychic Book
Everything® Reiki Book

Everything® Sex Signs Book, $9.95
Everything® Spells & Charms Book, 2nd Ed.
Everything® Tarot Book, 2nd Ed.
Everything® Toltec Wisdom Book
Everything® Wicca & Witchcraft Book, 2nd Ed.

PARENTING

Everything® Baby Names Book, 2nd Ed.
Everything® Baby Shower Book, 2nd Ed.
Everything® Baby Sign Language Book with DVD
Everything® Baby's First Year Book
Everything® Birthing Book
Everything® Breastfeeding Book
Everything® Father-to-Be Book
Everything® Father's First Year Book
Everything® Get Ready for Baby Book, 2nd Ed.
Everything® Get Your Baby to Sleep Book, $9.95
Everything® Getting Pregnant Book
Everything® Guide to Pregnancy Over 35
Everything® Guide to Raising a One-Year-Old
Everything® Guide to Raising a Two-Year-Old
Everything® Guide to Raising Adolescent Boys
Everything® Guide to Raising Adolescent Girls
Everything® Mother's First Year Book
Everything® Parent's Guide to Childhood Illnesses
Everything® Parent's Guide to Children and Divorce
Everything® Parent's Guide to Children with ADD/ADHD
Everything® Parent's Guide to Children with Asperger's
    Syndrome
Everything® Parent's Guide to Children with Anxiety
Everything® Parent's Guide to Children with Asthma
Everything® Parent's Guide to Children with Autism
Everything® Parent's Guide to Children with Bipolar Disorder
Everything® Parent's Guide to Children with Depression
Everything® Parent's Guide to Children with Dyslexia
Everything® Parent's Guide to Children with Juvenile Diabetes
Everything® Parent's Guide to Children with OCD
Everything® Parent's Guide to Positive Discipline
Everything® Parent's Guide to Raising Boys
Everything® Parent's Guide to Raising Girls
Everything® Parent's Guide to Raising Siblings
Everything® Parent's Guide to Raising Your
    Adopted Child
Everything® Parent's Guide to Sensory Integration Disorder
Everything® Parent's Guide to Tantrums
Everything® Parent's Guide to the Strong-Willed Child
Everything® Parenting a Teenager Book
Everything® Potty Training Book, $9.95
Everything® Pregnancy Book, 3rd Ed.
Everything® Pregnancy Fitness Book
Everything® Pregnancy Nutrition Book
Everything® Pregnancy Organizer, 2nd Ed., $16.95
Everything® Toddler Activities Book
Everything® Toddler Book
Everything® Tween Book
Everything® Twins, Triplets, and More Book

PETS

Everything® Aquarium Book
Everything® Boxer Book
Everything® Cat Book, 2nd Ed.
Everything® Chihuahua Book
Everything® Cooking for Dogs Book
Everything® Dachshund Book
Everything® Dog Book, 2nd Ed.
Everything® Dog Grooming Book

Everything® Dog Obedience Book
Everything® Dog Owner's Organizer, $16.95
Everything® Dog Training and Tricks Book
Everything® German Shepherd Book
Everything® Golden Retriever Book
Everything® Horse Book, 2nd Ed., $15.95
Everything® Horse Care Book
Everything® Horseback Riding Book
Everything® Labrador Retriever Book
Everything® Poodle Book
Everything® Pug Book
Everything® Puppy Book
Everything® Small Dogs Book
Everything® Tropical Fish Book
Everything® Yorkshire Terrier Book

REFERENCE

Everything® American Presidents Book
Everything® Blogging Book
Everything® Build Your Vocabulary Book, $9.95
Everything® Car Care Book
Everything® Classical Mythology Book
Everything® Da Vinci Book
Everything® Einstein Book
Everything® Enneagram Book
Everything® Etiquette Book, 2nd Ed.
Everything® Family Christmas Book, $15.95
Everything® Guide to C. S. Lewis & Narnia
Everything® Guide to Divorce, 2nd Ed., $15.95
Everything® Guide to Edgar Allan Poe
Everything® Guide to Understanding Philosophy
Everything® Inventions and Patents Book
Everything® Jacqueline Kennedy Onassis Book
Everything® John F. Kennedy Book
Everything® Mafia Book
Everything® Martin Luther King Jr. Book
Everything® Pirates Book
Everything® Private Investigation Book
Everything® Psychology Book
Everything® Public Speaking Book, $9.95
Everything® Shakespeare Book, 2nd Ed.

RELIGION

Everything® Angels Book
Everything® Bible Book
Everything® Bible Study Book with CD, $19.95
Everything® Buddhism Book
Everything® Catholicism Book
Everything® Christianity Book
Everything® Gnostic Gospels Book
Everything® Hinduism Book, $15.95
Everything® History of the Bible Book
Everything® Jesus Book
Everything® Jewish History & Heritage Book
Everything® Judaism Book
Everything® Kabbalah Book
Everything® Koran Book
Everything® Mary Book
Everything® Mary Magdalene Book
Everything® Prayer Book

Everything® Saints Book, 2nd Ed.
Everything® Torah Book
Everything® Understanding Islam Book
Everything® Women of the Bible Book
Everything® World's Religions Book

SCHOOL & CAREERS

Everything® Career Tests Book
Everything® College Major Test Book
Everything® College Survival Book, 2nd Ed.
Everything® Cover Letter Book, 2nd Ed.
Everything® Filmmaking Book
Everything® Get-a-Job Book, 2nd Ed.
Everything® Guide to Being a Paralegal
Everything® Guide to Being a Personal Trainer
Everything® Guide to Being a Real Estate Agent
Everything® Guide to Being a Sales Rep
Everything® Guide to Being an Event Planner
Everything® Guide to Careers in Health Care
Everything® Guide to Careers in Law Enforcement
Everything® Guide to Government Jobs
Everything® Guide to Starting and Running a Catering
   Business
Everything® Guide to Starting and Running a Restaurant
**Everything® Guide to Starting and Running
   a Retail Store**
Everything® Job Interview Book, 2nd Ed.
Everything® New Nurse Book
Everything® New Teacher Book
Everything® Paying for College Book
Everything® Practice Interview Book
Everything® Resume Book, 3rd Ed.
Everything® Study Book

SELF-HELP

Everything® Body Language Book
Everything® Dating Book, 2nd Ed.
Everything® Great Sex Book
**Everything® Guide to Caring for Aging Parents,
   $15.95**
Everything® Self-Esteem Book
Everything® Self-Hypnosis Book, $9.95
Everything® Tantric Sex Book

SPORTS & FITNESS

Everything® Easy Fitness Book
Everything® Fishing Book
Everything® Guide to Weight Training, $15.95
Everything® Krav Maga for Fitness Book
Everything® Running Book, 2nd Ed.
Everything® Triathlon Training Book, $15.95

TRAVEL

Everything® Family Guide to Coastal Florida
Everything® Family Guide to Cruise Vacations
Everything® Family Guide to Hawaii
Everything® Family Guide to Las Vegas, 2nd Ed.
Everything® Family Guide to Mexico
Everything® Family Guide to New England, 2nd Ed.

Everything® Family Guide to New York City, 3rd Ed.
**Everything® Family Guide to Northern California
   and Lake Tahoe**
Everything® Family Guide to RV Travel & Campgrounds
Everything® Family Guide to the Caribbean
Everything® Family Guide to the Disneyland® Resort, California
   Adventure®, Universal Studios®, and the Anaheim
   Area, 2nd Ed.
Everything® Family Guide to the Walt Disney World Resort®,
   Universal Studios®, and Greater Orlando, 5th Ed.
Everything® Family Guide to Timeshares
Everything® Family Guide to Washington D.C., 2nd Ed.

WEDDINGS

Everything® Bachelorette Party Book, $9.95
Everything® Bridesmaid Book, $9.95
Everything® Destination Wedding Book
Everything® Father of the Bride Book, $9.95
Everything® Green Wedding Book, $15.95
Everything® Groom Book, $9.95
Everything® Jewish Wedding Book, 2nd Ed., $15.95
Everything® Mother of the Bride Book, $9.95
Everything® Outdoor Wedding Book
Everything® Wedding Book, 3rd Ed.
Everything® Wedding Checklist, $9.95
Everything® Wedding Etiquette Book, $9.95
Everything® Wedding Organizer, 2nd Ed., $16.95
Everything® Wedding Shower Book, $9.95
Everything® Wedding Vows Book, 3rd Ed., $9.95
Everything® Wedding Workout Book
Everything® Weddings on a Budget Book, 2nd Ed., $9.95

WRITING

Everything® Creative Writing Book
Everything® Get Published Book, 2nd Ed.
Everything® Grammar and Style Book, 2nd Ed.
Everything® Guide to Magazine Writing
Everything® Guide to Writing a Book Proposal
Everything® Guide to Writing a Novel
Everything® Guide to Writing Children's Books
Everything® Guide to Writing Copy
Everything® Guide to Writing Graphic Novels
Everything® Guide to Writing Research Papers
Everything® Guide to Writing a Romance Novel, $15.95
Everything® Improve Your Writing Book, 2nd Ed.
Everything® Writing Poetry Book